THE COMPLETE CANDIDA FREE

COOKBOOK

100 Quick and Easy Delicious Recpes Fight Yeast & Candida

HOPE M. STITH

TABLE OF CONTENT

INTRODUCTION

Overgrowth of Candida can subtly impair your health by resulting in bloating, brain fog, skin problems, exhaustion, and more. Millions of people worldwide suffer with this common fungal imbalance, yet finding a solution can be difficult and daunting. This cookbook was created to help you combat Candida by providing you with clarity, taste, and sustenance.

More than just a set of recipes, "The Complete Candida Free Cookbook" is your go-to kitchen partner as you work to regain your energy, lower inflammation, and restore equilibrium, one delectable meal at a time.

WHAT YOU'LL FIND INSIDE

This book is thoughtfully organized to give you easy access to healing foods in every category. Whether you're craving a light bite or a hearty dinner, we've got you covered:

1. **Fresh & Healing Salads**
   Crisp, colorful, and packed with antifungal and detoxifying ingredients. These salads are designed to nourish your gut, support digestion, and keep your meals vibrant.
2. **Candida-Safe Soups & Broths**
   Soothing, warming, and deeply satisfying, these soups are made with immune-boosting herbs, low-starch vegetables, and healing broths to gently support your recovery.
3. **Low-Carb Breakfasts**
   Start your day strong with high-protein, low-sugar recipes that fuel your body without feeding yeast. Think egg bakes, chia bowls, and veggie-packed creations.
4. **Clean Proteins & Main Dishes**
   Savor robust meals featuring lean meats, wild fish, and plant-based proteins. These mains are rich in flavor but free from common Candida triggers like gluten, sugar, and dairy.

NWHY THIS COOKBOOK WORKS

Each of the 100 recipes is carefully crafted to meet Candida-diet guidelines—focusing on low-sugar, anti-inflammatory, gut-healing foods. They're not only Candida-safe, but also:

- Quick & Easy to Prepare
- Balanced with Macros for Energy and Healing k
- Family-Friendly & Flavor-Packed
- Customizable for Vegan, Paleo, and Keto Diets

You won't feel like you're missing out—in fact, you'll be amazed at how satisfying Candida-friendly meals can be.

⬜ WHAT YOU Can EAT VS WHAT YOU Can't EAT

The Candida diet supports your body with anti-inflammatory, healing elements while starving harmful yeast by eliminating the foods that feed it. The fight against Candida begins in your kitchen.

Foods You Can Eat

- Non-starchy vegetables (zucchini, spinach, cauliflower, broccoli)
- Low-sugar fruits (green apples, berries, lemons, avocado)
- Lean proteins (chicken, turkey, eggs, wild-caught fish)
- Healthy fats (olive oil, coconut oil, flaxseeds, avocados)
- Fermented foods (sauerkraut, kimchi, unsweetened coconut yogurt)
- Herbs & spices (garlic, turmeric, oregano, basil)
- Gluten-free grains (quinoa, buckwheat, millet—in moderation)

⬜ Foods You Can't Eat

- ✘ Refined sugars (white sugar, syrups, artificial sweeteners)
- ✘ Gluten & wheat products (bread, pasta, pastries)
- ✘ Alcohol & caffeine
- ✘ Processed foods & preservatives
- ✘ High-sugar fruits (bananas, grapes, mangoes, pineapples)
- ✘ Moldy foods (cheese, mushrooms, peanuts)
- ✘ Dairy (especially lactose-rich varieties)

BENEFITS OF FOLLOWING A CANDIDA-FREE DIET

Choosing Candida-safe recipes doesn't just help control yeast—it can transform your whole health. Here's what you may experience:

- ✓ Increased energy and reduced fatigue
- ✓ Improved digestion and relief from bloating or gas
- ✓ Clearer skin and reduction in acne or rashes
- ✓ Better focus and mental clarity
- ✓ Stronger immunity and fewer infections
- ✓ Balanced hormones and reduced sugar cravings
- ✓ Improved mood and reduced anxiety or brain fog

TIPS & TRICKS FOR CANDIDA COOKING SUCCESS

- **Meal Prep Weekly:** Planning ahead reduces temptation and ensures you stay on track.
- **Flavor with Herbs:** Use garlic, ginger, oregano, and cinnamon to boost antifungal power naturally.
- **Read Labels Carefully:** Many packaged foods contain hidden sugars and yeast.
- **Hydration is Key:** Drink lemon water and herbal teas to flush toxins.
- **Introduce Ferments Slowly:** Support your gut, but start with small servings of probiotic foods.
- **Track Your Reactions:** Everyone heals at a different pace—adjust ingredients as needed.

ADVANTAGES OF THIS COOKBOOK

Why choose The Complete Candida Free Cookbook? Because it makes healing simple, realistic, and flavorful. Here's what makes this book stand out:

- 100 Curated Recipes for every meal type—from breakfast to dinner
- Quick and Easy Instructions that fit any lifestyle
- Versatile for Different Diets (Paleo, Low-Carb, Dairy-Free, Vegan Options)
- No Fancy Equipment Needed—just whole foods and a basic kitchen
- Educational Guidance to help you understand your healing journey
- Family-Friendly Recipes even picky eaters will enjoy

CONCLUSION

Candida overgrowth doesn't have to control your life. With The Complete Candida Free Cookbook, you'll not only eliminate the yeast-feeding foods but also fall in love with healing meals that are vibrant, energizing, and delicious. Whether you're just starting your Candida journey or looking for new inspiration, this cookbook is your trusted companion.

Every recipe is a step toward:

- Balance
- Vitality
- Wellness

Your body has the power to heal—let food be your medicine. Let's get cooking.

1. COCONUT CHIA PUDDING

Prep Time: 5 Mins

Total Time: 4 Hrs (Chill Time)

Servings: 2

Ingredients

- 1 cup of full-fat coconut milk (unsweetened)
- 3 tbsp chia seeds
- ½tsp vanilla extract (non-compulsory, alcohol-free)
- Stevia or monk fruit sweetener (non-compulsory, +)
- A pinch of cinnamon (non-compulsory)

Instructions

1. Mix the coconut milk, chia seeds, sugar, and vanilla in a small dish or container.
2. After ten min, mix one more to disperse any clumps.
3. Cover and place in the refrigerator for at least four hours or overnight.
4. Before serving, stir and, if you'd like, sprinkle some unsweetened coconut flakes on top.

Notes

- ✓ Always use full-fat canned coconut milk for the best texture.
- ✓ You can flavor it with a pinch of cardamom or nutmeg for variation.

Nutrition Info (Per Serving)

- Calories: 240
- Fat: 22g
- Carbs: 6g
- Fiber: 5g
- Sugar: 1g
- Protein: 4g

2. SCRAMBLED EGGS WITH SPINACH

Prep Time: 3 Mins

Cook Time: 5 Mins

Total Time: 8 Mins

Servings: 1

Ingredients

- 2 large eggs
- ½cup of fresh spinach, chop-up
- 1 tbsp coconut oil or avocado oil
- Pinch of sea salt
- Pinch of black pepper

Instructions

1. Whisk together the eggs, salt, and pepper in a small bowl.
2. In a cast-iron or nonstick skillet, heat the oil over medium heat.
3. Add the spinach and cook until it wilts about 1 minute.
4. After adding the eggs to the skillet, cook them while stirring gently until they are set and scrambled.
5. Serve right away.

Notes

- ✓ Add herbs like dill, parsley, or chives for extra flavor.
- ✓ You can swap spinach for kale or arugula if preferred.

Nutrition Info (Per Serving)

- Calories: 220
- Fat: 18g
- Carbs: 2g
- Fiber: 1g
- Sugar: 0g
- Protein: 14g

3. ALMOND FLOUR Pancakes (No Sugar)

Prep Time: 5 Mins

Cook Time: 10 Mins

Total Time: 15 Mins

Servings: 2

Ingredients

- 1 cup of almond flour
- 2 large eggs
- 2 tbsp unsweetened almond milk
- ½tsp baking soda
- ½tsp apple cider vinegar
- ½tsp cinnamon (non-compulsory)
- Pinch of salt
- Coconut oil for cooking

Instructions

1. Mix the almond flour, baking soda, salt, and cinnamon in a medium-sized bowl.
2. Beat the eggs, almond milk, and apple cider vinegar in a separate bowl.
3. Mix the dry and wet components to make a batter.
4. In a pan, heat the coconut oil over medium-low heat.
5. Fill the skillet with two to three tbsp of batter for every pancake.
6. Cook until golden brown, 2 to 3 min per side.

Notes

- ✓ Simmer pancakes on medium-low to avoid burning.
- ✓ Serve with a dollop of coconut cream or a sprinkle of cinnamon.

Nutrition Info (Per Serving)

- Calories: 280
- Fat: 23g
- Carbs: 8g
- Fiber: 4g
- Sugar: 1g
- Protein: 12g

4. AVOCADO EGG BOATS

Prep Time: 5 Mins

Cook Time: 15 Mins

Total Time: 20 Mins

Servings: 2

Ingredients

- 1 ripe avocado
- 2 small eggs
- Salt and pepper+
- Paprika or chili flakes (non-compulsory)
- Fresh herbs for garnish (non-compulsory)

Instructions

1. Turn the oven on to 400°F or 200°C.
2. Halve the avocado and scoop out the pit.
3. Scoop out a little more flesh to make room for the egg.
4. Place avocado halves snugly in a baking dish.
5. Crack one egg into every avocado half.
6. Season with salt, pepper, and paprika.
7. Bake for 12–15 min until eggs are cooked to your liking.
8. Garnish with fresh herbs if desired.

Notes

✓ If your avocado halves are wobbly, nestle them into a small ramekin or use crumpled foil to steady them.
✓ Try topping with a sprinkle of nutritional yeast for a "cheesy" flavor without dairy.

Nutrition Info (Per Serving)

- Calories: 190
- Fat: 16g
- Carbs: 6g
- Fiber: 5g
- Sugar: 0g
- Protein: 7g

5. ZUCCHINI HASH BROWNS

Prep Time: 10 Mins

Cook Time: 10 Mins

Total Time: 20 Mins

Servings: 2

Ingredients

- 2 medium zucchinis, finely grated
- 1 large egg

- 2 tbsp coconut flour
- ½tsp sea salt
- ¼ tsp black pepper
- 1 tbsp coconut oil (for frying)

Instructions

1. Using a fresh cloth, grate the zucchini and wring out as much liquid as possible.
2. Mix the zucchini, egg, coconut flour, salt, and pepper in a bowl. Stir well.
3. In a pan, heat the coconut oil over medium heat.
4. Scoop out tiny amounts of the mixture in the pan and press them into patties.
5. Cook until golden brown and crispy, approximately 3 to 4 min per side.
6. Warm up and serve.

Notes

✓ Removing the moisture from the zucchini is key to crispy hash browns.
✓ You can add herbs like parsley or chives for extra flavor.

Nutrition Info (Per Serving)

- Calories: 190
- Fat: 14g
- Carbs: 7g
- Fiber: 3g
- Sugar: 3g
- Protein: 7g

6. COCONUT Yogurt With Flaxseeds

Total Time: 2 Mins

Servings: 1

Ingredients

- ¾ cup of unsweetened coconut yogurt (dairy-free)
- 1 tbsp ground flaxseeds
- Non-compulsory: cinnamon or stevia for extra flavor

Instructions

1. In a dish, scoop out the coconut yogurt.
2. Add ground flaxseeds and stir until thoroughly mixed.
3. Add a small pinch of stevia or cinnamon, if desired.
4. Enjoy right now, or let it thicken by chilling it for ten minutes.

Notes

- ✓ Use a brand of coconut yogurt with no added sugars or gums.
- ✓ Flaxseeds boost fiber and support digestion.

Nutrition Info (Per Serving)

- ↓ Calories: 220
- ↓ Fat: 18g
- ↓ Carbs: 6g
- ↓ Fiber: 5g
- ↓ Sugar: 1g
- ↓ Protein: 3g

7. CAULIFLOWER "OATMEAL"

Prep Time: 5 Mins

Cook Time: 10 Mins

Total Time: 15 Mins

Servings: 2

Ingredients

- 2 cups of cauliflower rice (fresh or frozen)
- ¾ cup of full-fat coconut milk
- 1 tbsp ground flaxseeds
- 1 tbsp coconut flakes (unsweetened)
- ½tsp cinnamon
- Stevia or monk fruit+

Instructions

1. Put the coconut milk and cauliflower rice in a small saucepan.
2. Cook until the cauliflower is tender, about 5 to 7 minutes, over medium heat.
3. Add the coconut flakes, cinnamon, flaxseeds, and sweetener and stir.
4. Simmer until thickened, 2 to 3 min more.
5. Warm up and serve.

Notes

- ✓ For extra texture, stir in chop-up walnuts or pecans (if tolerated).
- ✓ You can blend the cauliflower slightly for a smoother "porridge" feel.

Nutrition Info (Per Serving)

- Calories: 180
- Fat: 14g
- Carbs: 7g
- Fiber: 4g
- Sugar: 2g
- Protein: 4g

8. COLLAGEN PROTEIN SMOOTHIE (NO FRUIT)

Total Time: 3 Mins

Servings: 1

Ingredients

- 1 scoop unflavored collagen peptides
- 1 cup of unsweetened almond milk (or coconut milk)
- 1 tbsp MCT oil or coconut oil
- ½tsp cinnamon
- A few drops of stevia or monk fruit (non-compulsory)
- Ice cubes (non-compulsory, for texture)

Instructions

1. Mix almond milk, collagen peptides, MCT oil, cinnamon, and sweetener in a blender.
2. Mix until frothy and smooth.
3. Add ice cubes and mix once more for a while if desired.
4. Transfer to a glass and savor.

Notes

- ✓ This smoothie is great for gut healing and skin support.
- ✓ You can add a tsp of unsweetened cocoa powder for a chocolatey version.

Nutrition Info (Per Serving)

- Calories: 150
- Fat: 10g
- Carbs: 2g
- Fiber: 1g
- Sugar: 0g
- Protein: 13g

9. SAVORY BREAKFAST MUFFINS (ALMOND OR COCONUT FLOUR)

Prep Time: 10 Mins

Cook Time: 20 Mins

Total Time: 30 Mins

Servings: 6

Ingredients

- 1 cup of almond flour (or ½cup of coconut flour)
- 4 large eggs
- ¼ cup of unsweetened almond milk or coconut milk
- ¼ cup of chop-up spinach
- ¼ cup of diced onions
- ¼ tsp baking soda
- ¼ tsp sea salt
- ¼ tsp black pepper
- 1 tbsp coconut oil (melted)

Instructions

1. Set the oven temperature to 175°C (350°F).
2. Grease a muffin tray thoroughly or line it with silicone liners.
3. Whisk the eggs, coconut oil, and almond milk in a bowl.
4. Add baking soda, salt, pepper, and almond flour and stir.
5. Add chop-up onions and spinach and fold.
6. Evenly fill muffin cups with batter.
7. Muffins should be firm and begin turning brown after 18 to 20 minutes of baking.
8. Before taking it out of the pan, let it cool.

Notes

- ✓ Add cooked turkey bacon bits or herbs like parsley for more flavor.
- ✓ Muffins can be frozen and reheated for quick breakfasts.

Nutrition Info (Per Muffin):

- ↓ Calories: 150
- ↓ Fat: 12g
- ↓ Carbs: 4g
- ↓ Fiber: 2g

- Sugar: 1g
- Protein: 7g

10. MUSHROOM AND ONION OMELET

Prep Time: 5 Mins

Cook Time: 7 Mins

Total Time: 12 Mins

Servings: 1

Ingredients

- 2 large eggs
- ¼ cup of Sliced mushrooms
- 2 tbsp diced onion
- 1 tbsp coconut oil or avocado oil
- Pinch of sea salt
- Pinch of black pepper

Instructions

1. Beat the eggs with salt and pepper in a bowl.
2. In a skillet, heat the oil over medium heat.
3. Sauté the onions and mushrooms for three to four minutes or until tender.
4. Evenly distribute the beaten eggs over the vegetables by tilting the pan.
5. Cook until the bottom is set, 2 to 3 min.
6. Cook the omelet for one more minute after carefully flipping or folding it.
7. Transfer to a platter and proceed to serve.

Notes

- ✓ Feel free to add herbs like thyme or parsley to the mushroom mix.
- ✓ You can add a sprinkle of nutritional yeast for a cheesy flavor without dairy.

Nutrition Info (Per Serving)

- Calories: 220
- Fat: 17g
- Carbs: 3g
- Fiber: 1g
- Sugar: 1g
- Protein: 12g

11. GREEN DETOX SMOOTHIE (WITH KALE AND CUCUMBER)

Total Time: 5 Mins

Servings: 1

Ingredients

- 1 cup of kale leaves (stems removed)
- ½cucumber, Sliced
- ½avocado
- 1 tbsp lemon juice
- ½tsp fresh finely grated ginger
- 1 cup of water or coconut water (unsweetened)
- Ice cubes (non-compulsory)

Instructions

1. Mix the kale, cucumber, avocado, lemon juice, ginger, and water in a blender.
2. Blend until the mixture is absolutely smooth.
3. If you want it cooler, add ice cubes and mix once more.
4. Enjoy it fresh after pouring it into a glass.

Notes

- ✓ You can add a few mint leaves for extra freshness.
- ✓ Use coconut water only if you tolerate a little natural sugar.

Nutrition Info (Per Serving)

- Calories: 140
- Fat: 10
- Carbs: 8g
- Fiber: 5g
- Sugar: 2g
- Protein: 3g

12. COCONUT Milk Smoothie With Cinnamon

Total Time: 3 Mins

Servings: 1

Ingredients

- 1 cup of full-fat coconut milk
- 1 tbsp chia seeds
- ½tsp ground cinnamon
- ½tsp vanilla extract (alcohol-free, non-compulsory)
- Stevia or monk fruit drops (non-compulsory)
- Ice cubes (non-compulsory)

Instructions

1. Mix coconut milk, chia seeds, cinnamon, vanilla, and sweetener in a blender.
2. Blend until smooth and well indefinitely grated.
3. For a thicker, colder texture, add ice cubes.
4. Pour into a glass, then take a leisurely drink.

Notes

✓ After blending, let it sit for a few minutes to thicken it slightly.
✓ Sprinkle extra cinnamon on top before serving for a cozy touch.

Nutrition Info (Per Serving)

- Calories: 210
- Fat: 19g
- Carbs: 5g
- Fiber: 3g
- Sugar: 1g
- Protein: 3g

13. TURMERIC CAULIFLOWER RICE BOWL

Prep Time: 10 Mins

Cook Time: 10 Mins

Total Time: 20 Mins

Servings: 2

Ingredients

- 2 cup of cauliflower rice
- 1 tbsp coconut oil

- ½tsp turmeric powder
- ¼ tsp cumin powder
- ¼ tsp sea salt
- ⅛ tsp black pepper
- 1 tbsp fresh parsley or cilantro (non-compulsory)

Instructions

1. In a pan, heat the coconut oil over medium heat.
2. Sauté the cauliflower rice for two to three min.
3. Add the cumin, turmeric, salt, and pepper and stir.
4. Cook the cauliflower for 5 to 7 min, stirring now and again, until it is soft.
5. Before serving, garnish with chop-up cilantro or parsley.

Notes

- ✓ Add cooked chicken or a fried egg to a more complete meal.
- ✓ Fresh turmeric root can be used instead of powder for extra flavor and benefits.

Nutrition Info (Per Serving)

- Calories: 130
- Fat: 10g
- Carbs: 6g
- Fiber: 3g
- Sugar: 2g
- Protein: 3g

14. COCONUT FLOUR WAFFLES (UNSWEETENED)

Prep Time: 5 Mins

Cook Time: 8 Mins

Total Time: 13 Mins

Servings: 2

Ingredients

- ⅓ cup of coconut flour
- 3 large eggs
- ¼ cup of unsweetened coconut milk
- 1 tbsp coconut oil, melted
- ½tsp baking powder

- ½tsp cinnamon (non-compulsory)
- Pinch of sea salt

Instructions

1. Follow the manufacturer's directions to preheat the waffle maker.
2. Whisk the eggs, coconut milk, and coconut oil in a bowl.
3. Add baking powder, salt, cinnamon, and coconut flour. Mix to blend.
4. For the batter to thicken, let it sit for two to three min.
5. Fill the waffle machine with batter, then cook it until it's crisp and golden brown.
6. Warm up and serve.

Notes

- ✓ These waffles freeze well — reheat them in a toaster.
- ✓ Top with a dollop of coconut cream or a sprinkle of cinnamon.

Nutrition Info (Per Waffle):

- Calories: 180
- Fat: 14g
- Carbs: 6g
- Fiber: 4g
- Sugar: 1
- Protein: 7g

15. BROCCOLI AND CHEDDAR FRITTATA

Prep Time: 7 Mins

Cook Time: 18 Mins

Total Time: 25 Mins

Servings: 4

Ingredients

- 6 large eggs
- 1 cup of small broccoli florets (lightly steamed)
- ½cup of shredded organic cheddar cheese (or a dairy-free alternative)
- ¼ cup of coconut milk (non-compulsory for creaminess)
- ½tsp sea salt
- ¼ tsp black pepper
- 1 tbsp avocado oil (for greasing the pan)

Instructions

1. Turn the oven on to 375°F, or 190°C.
2. Apply avocado oil to a cast iron pan or small baking dish.
3. Whisk together eggs, salt, pepper, and coconut milk, if using, in a bowl.
4. Evenly distribute the broccoli in the dish and top with cheese.
5. Over the top, pour the egg mixture.
6. Bake until the middle is firm, 18 to 20 min.
7. Before slicing, allow it to cool somewhat.

Notes

✓ You can substitute broccoli for spinach, zucchini, or mushrooms.
✓ Use a sharp cheddar for the most flavor, if including dairy.

Nutrition Info (Per Serving)

- Calories: 210
- Fat: 16g
- Carbs: 4g
- Fiber: 2g
- Sugar: 1g
- Protein: 12g

=

16. SARDINES AND AVOCADO TOAST (ON ALMOND BREAD)

Prep Time: 5 Mins

Cook Time: 2 Mins (To Toast The Bread)

Total Time: 7 Mins

Servings: 1

Ingredients

- 1 slice almond flour bread
- ½ripe avocado
- 1 can sardines (packed in water or olive oil), drained
- ½tbsp lemon juice
- Pinch of sea salt
- Pinch of black pepper
- Red pepper flakes (non-compulsory)

Instructions

1. The piece of almond bread should be gently crunchy after toasting.
2. Add salt, pepper, and lemon juice to the avocado and mash it.
3. Cover the bread with mashed avocado.
4. If desired, garnish with red pepper flakes and sardines.
5. Serve right away.

Notes

✓ Sardines are rich in omega-3s and very gut-friendly.
✓ For variety, add Sliced cucumber or radish on top.

Nutrition Info (Per Serving)

- Calories: 320
- Fat: 22g
- Carbs: 8g
- Fiber: 5g
- Sugar: 1g
- Protein: 18g

17. LEMON GINGER DETOX TEA

Prep Time: 5 Mins

Cook Time: 10 Mins

Total Time: 15 Mins

Servings: 2

Ingredients

- 2 cup of water
- 1-inch piece of fresh ginger, Sliced
- 1 tbsp fresh lemon juice
- Non-compulsory: a few drops of liquid stevia

Instructions

1. In a small saucepan, bring water and ginger slices to a simmer.
2. Simmer for ten min or so.
3. Strain into mugs after removing from the heat.
4. Add the fresh lemon juice and stir.
5. If you like a touch of sweetness, add stevia.

Notes

- ✓ For an extra anti-inflammatory boost, add a pinch of turmeric.
- ✓ Best enjoyed warm on an empty stomach in the morning.

Nutrition Info (Per Serving)

- ↓ Calories: 5
- ↓ Carbs: 1g

18. PUMPKIN SEED PORRIDGE

Prep Time: 5 Mins

Cook Time: 7 Mins

Total Time: 12 Mins

Servings: 1

Ingredients

- ¼ cup of raw pumpkin seeds
- 1 tbsp chia seeds
- 1 tbsp flaxseeds
- ¾ cup of unsweetened almond milk
- ½tsp cinnamon
- Stevia or monk fruit+

Instructions

1. Grind flaxseeds, chia, and pumpkin seeds into a coarse meal in a food processor.
2. Add the cinnamon and almond milk to a small saucepan.
3. Gently heat, stirring frequently, until thickened, 5 to 7 min.
4. Serve warm, sweetened+.

Notes

- ✓ You can top it with a few extra pumpkin seeds for crunch.
- ✓ Excellent source of zinc and healthy fats.

Nutrition Info (Per Serving)

- ↓ Calories: 260
- ↓ Fat: 20g
- ↓ Carbs: 8g
- ↓ Fiber: 5g

- Sugar: 1g
- Protein: 10g

19. BONE BROTH BREAKFAST SOUP

Prep Time: 5 Mins

Cook Time: 15 Mins

Total Time: 20 Mins

Servings: 2

Ingredients

- 2 cups of high-quality bone broth (chicken or beef)
- ½cup of diced zucchini
- ½cup of chop-up spinach
- 1 tbsp coconut aminos
- 1 tbsp fresh parsley
- 1 tsp finely grated ginger
- ¼ tsp sea salt (non-compulsory)

Instructions

1. In a saucepan, bring bone broth to low heat.
2. Cook the zucchini for five minutes or until it begins to soften.
3. Add the ginger, parsley, coconut aminos, and spinach and stir.
4. Simmer for a further two to three min.
5. If necessary, taste and adjust the seasoning. Warm up and serve.

Notes

- ✓ It is very healing for the gut and rich in collagen.
- ✓ You can add shredded cooked chicken for extra protein.

Nutrition Info (Per Serving)

- Calories: 120
- Fat: 5g
- Carbs: 3g
- Fiber: 1g
- Sugar: 1g
- Protein: 15g

20. PALEO BREAKFAST SAUSAGE PATTIES

Prep Time: 10 Mins

Cook Time: 10 Mins

Total Time: 20 Mins

Servings: 4

Ingredients

- 1 lb ground turkey or ground pork
- 1 tsp dried sage
- ½tsp garlic powder
- ½tsp onion powder
- ½tsp sea salt
- ¼ tsp black pepper
- ⅛ tsp crushed red pepper flakes (non-compulsory)
- 1 tbsp coconut oil (for frying)

Instructions

1. Mix the ingredients and the beef in a bowl.
2. Form into tiny, flat patties after thoroughly mixing.
3. In a pan, heat the coconut oil over medium heat.
4. Cook patties until golden brown and cooked through, about 4 to 5 min every side.
5. Warm up and serve.

Notes

- ✓ You can double the batch and freeze cooked patties for easy breakfasts.
- ✓ Great served with sautéed greens or avocado.

Nutrition Info (Per Serving - 2 patties):

- Calories: 220
- Fat: 15g
- Carbs: 1g
- Protein: 20g

21. LEMON HERB GRILLED CHICKEN SALAD

Prep Time: 10 Mins

Cook Time: 15 Mins

Total Time: 25 Mins

Servings: 2

Ingredients

- 2 boneless, skinless chicken breasts
- 2 tbsp olive oil
- 2 tbsp lemon juice
- 1 tsp dried oregano
- 1 tsp garlic powder
- Salt and pepper,+
- 4 cups of mixed greens (spinach, arugula, lettuce)
- ½cucumber, Sliced
- ½avocado, Sliced
- ¼ red onion, thinly Sliced

Instructions

1. Mix oil, lemon juice, oregano, garlic powder, salt, and pepper.
2. Coat them in a bowl of chicken breasts with the marinade and let them sit for 10 to 15 minutes.
3. Set a grill or grill pan over medium-high heat.
4. After 6 to 8 min on every side of the grill, the chicken should be cooked thoroughly, with an internal temperature of 165°F (74°C).
5. Slice the chicken once it has rested for a few min.
6. Toss in the mixed greens, cucumber, avocado, and red onion.
7. Top with grilled chicken pieces and, if desired, drizzle with additional olive oil and lemon juice.

Notes

- ✓ For extra flavor, marinate chicken for up to 1 hr.
- ✓ Add pumpkin seeds for extra crunch.

Nutrition Info (Per Serving)

- Calories: 360
- Fat: 22g
- Carbs: 8g
- Fiber: 5g
- Sugar: 2g
- Protein: 32g

22. CAULIFLOWER FRIED "RICE"

Prep Time: 10 Mins

Cook Time: 10 Mins

Total Time: 20 Mins

Servings: 3

Ingredients

- 1 medium head of cauliflower, riced
- 2 tbsp coconut oil
- 2 cloves garlic, chop-up
- ½cup of diced carrots
- ½cup of peas (non-compulsory, if tolerated)
- 2 eggs, lightly beaten
- 2 tbsp coconut aminos (or tamari if tolerated)
- 2 green onions, Sliced
- Salt and pepper,+

Instructions

1. In a food processor, pulse the cauliflower florets until they have the consistency of rice.
2. In a large pan, heat the coconut oil over medium heat.
3. Sauté the carrots and garlic for two to three min.
4. After pushing the veggies to one side of the skillet, add the beaten eggs and scramble until they are cooked.
5. Stir everything together after adding the riced cauliflower and coconut aminos.
6. Cook the cauliflower until it is soft but not mushy, stirring regularly, about 5 to 7 min.
7. Season with salt and pepper, stir in green onions and serve hot.

Notes

- ✓ You can add diced cooked chicken or shrimp for a protein boost.
- ✓ Frozen pre-riced cauliflower works excellent for a quicker version.

Nutrition Info (Per Serving)

- Calories: 160
- Fat: 10g
- Carbs: 10g

- Fiber: 4g
- Sugar: 3g
- Protein: 7g

23. ROASTED VEGETABLE BUDDHA BOWL

Prep Time: 15 Mins

Cook Time: 25 Mins

Total Time: 40 Mins

Servings: 2

Ingredients

- 1 small sweet potato, diced
- 1 cup of broccoli florets
- 1 red bell pepper, chop up
- 2 tbsp olive oil
- ½tsp smoked paprika
- Salt and pepper,+
- 2 cups of mixed greens (like spinach or arugula)
- ½avocado, Sliced
- 2 tbsp pumpkin seeds (non-compulsory)
- Lemon wedges for serving

Instructions

1. Turn the oven on to 400°F or 200°C.
2. Add the smoked paprika, olive oil, salt, pepper, sweet potato, broccoli, and red bell pepper.
3. Arrange the veggies on a baking sheet and roast them for 20 to 25 min, tossing them halfway through until they are soft and crisp.
4. Mix mixed greens at the bottom of every bowl to construct.
5. Add slices of avocado, roasted veggies, and, if using, pumpkin seeds on top.
6. Before serving, drizzle everything with freshly squeezed lemon juice.

Notes

- ✓ Swap vegetables based on season — zucchini, asparagus, or cauliflower are great options.
- ✓ Add a sprinkle of hemp seeds for extra nutrition.

Nutrition Info (Per Serving)

- Calories: 300
- Fat: 20g
- Carbs: 22g
- Fiber: 7g
- Sugar: 5g
- Protein: 7g

24. GARLIC SHRIMP WITH ZOODLES

Prep Time: 10 Mins

Cook Time: 8 Mins

Total Time: 18 Mins

Servings: 2

Ingredients

- 2 medium zucchinis, spiralized into noodles
- ½lb shrimp, peeled and deveined
- 2 tbsp olive oil
- 3 cloves garlic, chop-up
- ¼ tsp crushed red pepper flakes (non-compulsory)
- 1 tbsp lemon juice
- Sea salt and black pepper,+
- Fresh parsley for garnish

Instructions

1. Heat 1 tbsp of olive oil in a large pan over medium heat.
2. Cook the shrimp for two to three minutes on every side, or until they are cooked through and pink. Could you remove them and set them aside?
3. Sauté the garlic in the skillet for 30 seconds after adding olive oil.
4. Add the zoodles and cook until they are barely soft, about 2 to 3 min.
5. Reintroduce the shrimp to the pan, add salt and pepper, and sprinkle with lemon juice.
6. Mix everything and add parsley as a garnish.

Notes

- ✓ Avoid overcooking the zoodles to keep them slightly crunchy.
- ✓ You can swap shrimp for scallops if you like.

Nutrition Info (Per Serving)

- Calories: 280
- Fat: 16g
- Carbs: 7g
- Fiber: 2g
- Sugar: 4g
- Protein: 26g

25. CUCUMBER AVOCADO GAZPACHO

Total Time: 10 Mins

Servings: 2

Ingredients

- 1 large cucumber, peeled and chop up
- 1 ripe avocado
- ¼ cup of fresh cilantro
- 1 tbsp lime juice
- ½cup of cold water
- 1 small garlic clove
- Sea salt and black pepper,+

Instructions

1. Mix the cucumber, avocado, cilantro, lime juice, water, and garlic in a blender.
2. Blend till creamy and smooth.
3. As needed, add salt and pepper.
4. Serve immediately, or chill for 20 minutes if you want it cold.

Notes

- ✓ Add a splash of more water if you prefer a thinner soup.
- ✓ Perfect for hot days and very hydrating!

Nutrition Info (Per Serving)

- Calories: 160
- Fat: 12g
- Carbs: 10g
- Fiber: 6g
- Sugar: 2g
- Protein: 3g

26. TURKEY LETTUCE WRAPS

Prep Time: 10 Mins

Cook Time: 10 Mins

Total Time: 20 Mins

Servings: 2

Ingredients

- ½lb ground turkey
- 1 tbsp coconut oil
- ¼ cup of diced onions
- 1 clove garlic, chop-up
- 1 tbsp coconut aminos
- 1 tsp ground ginger
- ½tsp sea salt
- 1 head butter lettuce or romaine leaves
- Non-compulsory toppings: Sliced green onions, sesame seeds

Instructions

1. In a pan over medium heat, warm the coconut oil.
2. Add garlic and onions, and cook for two to three min.
3. Cook the ground turkey till it turns golden brown.
4. Add ground ginger, coconut aminos, and salt and stir.
5. Decorate the turkey mixture after spooning it onto the lettuce leaves.

Notes

- ✓ These wraps are great for meal prep — keep the filling and lettuce separate until ready to eat.
- ✓ You can also substitute turkey with ground chicken.

Nutrition Info (Per Serving)

- Calories: 230
- Fat: 14g
- Carbs: 4g
- Fiber: 2g
- Sugar: 1g
- Protein: 22g

27. GRILLED SALMON WITH ASPARAGUS

Prep Time: 5 Mins

Cook Time: 12 Mins

Total Time: 17 Mins

Servings: 2

Ingredients

- 2 salmon fillets (about 6 oz every)
- 1 bunch asparagus, trimmed
- 2 tbsp olive oil
- 1 tbsp lemon juice
- 1 tsp dried dill (non-compulsory)
- Sea salt and black pepper,+

Instructions

1. Turn the heat up to medium-high on the grill or grill pan.
2. Add salt, pepper, and dill to the fish and asparagus after brushing them with olive oil.
3. Salmon should be cooked through after grilling for 4 to 5 min on every side.
4. Sauté asparagus for 5 to 7 min, tossing regularly until tender.
5. Before serving, pour lemon juice over everything.

Notes

- ✓ Use foil if you're worried about salmon sticking to the grill.
- ✓ Fresh dill or parsley brightens up the dish!

Nutrition Info (Per Serving)

- Calories: 370
- Fat: 24g
- Carbs: 5g
- Fiber: 2g
- Sugar: 2g
- Protein: 32g

28. COCONUT CURRY CHICKEN SOUP

Prep Time: 10 Mins

Cook Time: 20 Mins

Total Time: 30 Mins

Servings: 4

Ingredients

- 1 tbsp coconut oil
- ½cup of diced onions
- 2 cloves garlic, chop-up
- 1 tbsp finely grated ginger
- 1 tbsp curry powder
- 1 lb chicken breast, diced
- 4 cups of chicken bone broth
- 1 cup of full-fat coconut milk
- 1 cup of chop-up spinach
- 1 tbsp lime juice
- Sea salt and pepper,+

Instructions

1. Heat the coconut oil in a big saucepan over medium heat.
2. Sauté the ginger, garlic, and onions for three to four min.
3. Cook for one more minute after adding the curry powder.
4. Cook the diced chicken until it is no longer pink.
5. Add the coconut milk and bone broth, then bring to a boil.
6. Cook the spinach for three to five min or until it wilts.
7. Season with salt and pepper, stir in lime juice and serve.

Notes

- ✓ For extra spice, add a pinch of cayenne pepper.
- ✓ It works excellent with leftover shredded chicken, too!

Nutrition Info (Per Serving)

- Calories: 310
- Fat: 20g
- Carbs: 5g
- Fiber: 1g
- Sugar: 2g
- Protein: 26g

29. EGGPLANT LASAGNA (NO PASTA)

Prep Time: 15 Mins

Cook Time: 30 Mins

Total Time: 45 Mins

Servings: 4

Ingredients

- 2 medium eggplants, Sliced lengthwise into ¼-inch thick slices
- 1 tbsp olive oil
- 1 lb ground turkey or beef
- 1 cup of sugar-free marinara sauce
- ½tsp dried basil
- ½tsp dried oregano
- ½tsp garlic powder
- 1 cup of shredded mozzarella (or dairy-free cheese alternative)
- Sea salt and pepper,+

Instructions

1. Turn the oven on to 375°F, or 190°C.
2. After brushing them with olive oil, roast the eggplant slices for ten minutes or until tender.
3. In the meantime, brown ground beef or turkey in a pan.
4. Add the garlic powder, oregano, basil, marinara sauce, salt, and pepper and stir.
5. Arrange the cheese, meat sauce, and roasted eggplant in a baking dish.
6. Continue layering, and finish with cheese.
7. The cheese should be melted and bubbling after 20 min of baking.

Notes

- ✓ Let lasagna cool for 10 min before slicing to help it set.
- ✓ You can pre-salt eggplant slices to reduce moisture if desired.

Nutrition Info (Per Serving)

- Calories: 340
- Fat: 22g
- Carbs: 9g
- Fiber: 4g
- Sugar: 5g

+ Protein: 26g

30. ZUCCHINI NOODLE STIR FRY

Prep Time: 10 Mins

Cook Time: 8 Mins

Total Time: 18 Mins

Servings: 2

Ingredients

- 2 medium zucchinis, spiralized
- 1 tbsp coconut oil
- ½cup of Sliced bell peppers
- ½cup of Sliced mushrooms
- 1 clove garlic, chop-up
- 2 tbsp coconut aminos
- 1 tsp sesame seeds (non-compulsory)
- Sea salt and pepper,+

Instructions

1. Heat the coconut oil over medium-high heat in a large skillet or wok.
2. Stir-fry the garlic, bell peppers, and mushrooms for three to four min.
3. Toss with coconut aminos after adding the zucchini noodles.
4. Cook until the zoodles are soft but not mushy, about 2 to 3 minutes.
5. Add sesame seeds, if using, and season with salt and pepper.

Notes

✓ Keep the heat high and stir often to avoid soggy zoodles.
✓ You can add tofu, shrimp, or chicken for extra protein.

Nutrition Info (Per Serving)

+ Calories: 150
+ Fat: 10g
+ Carbs: 9g
+ Fiber: 3g
+ Sugar: 4g
+ Protein: 4g

31. CHICKEN BONE BROTH SOUP

Prep Time: 5 Mins

Cook Time: 15 Mins

Total Time: 20 Mins

Servings: 2

Ingredients

- 2 cups of chicken bone broth
- ½cup of shredded cooked chicken
- ½cup of diced zucchini
- ½cup of chop-up kale or spinach
- 1 clove garlic, chop-up
- 1 tbsp lemon juice
- Sea salt and pepper,+

Instructions

1. Bring the chicken bone broth to a simmer in a saucepan.
2. Add the garlic, kale, zucchini, and chicken shreds.
3. Simmer until the veggies are soft, 10 to 12 min.
4. Season with salt and pepper and stir in lemon juice.
5. Warm up and serve.

Notes

- ✓ Perfect for a healing, gut-friendly light meal.
- ✓ You can freeze portions for quick future meals.

Nutrition Info (Per Serving)

- Calories: 180
- Fat: 7g
- Carbs: 3g
- Fiber: 1g
- Sugar: 1g
- Protein: 24g

32. SPAGHETTI SQUASH WITH BASIL PESTO

Prep Time: 10 Mins

Cook Time: 40 Mins

Total Time: 50 Mins

Servings: 2

Ingredients

- 1 medium spaghetti squash
- 2 tbsp olive oil
- ½ cup of fresh basil leaves
- 2 tbsp pine nuts (or walnuts)
- 1 clove garlic
- 3 tbsp olive oil (for pesto)
- 2 tbsp nutritional yeast (non-compulsory)
- Salt and pepper,+

Instructions

1. Turn the oven on to 400°F or 200°C. After removing the seeds, cut the spaghetti squash in half lengthwise.
2. Place face down on a baking pan, drizzle with olive oil, and season with salt and pepper.
3. Roast until soft, 35 to 40 minutes. Allow it to cool somewhat, then use a fork to scrape the meat into "noodles."
4. As the squash roasts, prepare the pesto: Add the nutritional yeast, garlic, nuts, basil, olive oil, salt, and pepper and blend until smooth.
5. Serve the spaghetti squash strands warm after tossing them with pesto.

Notes

- ✓ Add grilled chicken or shrimp on top for a complete meal.
- ✓ Store leftover pesto in an airtight container in the fridge for up to 5 days.

Nutrition Info (Per Serving)

- ♦ Calories: 290
- ♦ Fat: 21g
- ♦ Carbs: 17g
- ♦ Fiber: 5g
- ♦ Sugar: 6g
- ♦ Protein: 5g

33. THAI COCONUT SOUP (TOM KHA GAI)

Prep Time: 10 Mins

Cook Time: 20 Mins

Total Time: 30 Mins

Servings: 3

Ingredients

- 1 tbsp coconut oil
- 2 cloves garlic, chop-up
- 1-inch piece of fresh ginger, Sliced
- 2 cup of chicken broth
- 1 cup of coconut milk (full-fat)
- 1 chicken breast, thinly Sliced
- 1 cup of mushrooms, Sliced
- 1 tbsp fish sauce
- 1 tbsp lime juice
- 2 kaffir lime leaves (non-compulsory)
- Fresh cilantro for garnish

Instructions

1. In a big saucepan, heat the coconut oil over medium heat. Ginger and garlic should be sautéed till aromatic.
2. Add the chicken pieces, mushrooms, coconut milk, and chicken broth.
3. Bring to a boil and cook until the chicken is cooked for about 10 to 12 minutes.
4. Add the lime juice, fish sauce, and, if using, the kaffir lime leaves.
5. Garnish with fresh cilantro and serve hot.

Notes

- ✓ You can substitute chicken with shrimp or tofu.
- ✓ For extra heat, add a few slices of Thai chili.

Nutrition Info (Per Serving)

- Calories: 310
- Fat: 22g
- Carbs: 7g
- Fiber: 1g
- Sugar: 2g

⬇ Protein: 20g

34. MEDITERRANEAN CAULIFLOWER SALAD

Prep Time: 15 Mins

Cook Time: 5 Mins

Total Time: 20 Mins

Servings: 4

Ingredients

- 1 medium head cauliflower, lightly chopped up or riced
- ½cup of cherry tomatoes, halved
- ¼ cucumber, diced
- ¼ red onion, diced
- 2 tbsp olive oil
- 1 tbsp lemon juice
- ¼ cup of black olives, Sliced
- 2 tbsp fresh parsley, chop-up
- Salt and pepper,+

Instructions

1. Cauliflower can be left raw for crunch or lightly steamed for three to five min (non-compulsory for a softer texture).
2. Add the cauliflower, tomatoes, cucumber, onion, and olives to a large bowl.
3. Pour lemon juice and olive oil over everything, then toss to coat.
4. Before serving, add fresh parsley over top and season with salt and pepper.

Notes

- ✓ Add crumbled feta (if tolerated) for extra Mediterranean flavor.
- ✓ Great as a side dish or a light lunch!

Nutrition Info (Per Serving)

- ⬇ Calories: 120
- ⬇ Fat: 9g
- ⬇ Carbs: 8g
- ⬇ Fiber: 3g
- ⬇ Sugar: 3g
- ⬇ Protein: 3g

35. WILD-CAUGHT TUNA SALAD (NO MAYO)

Total Time: 10 Mins

Servings: 2

Ingredients

- 1 can wild-caught tuna, drained
- 1 tbsp olive oil
- 1 tsp Dijon mustard (non-compulsory)
- ½avocado, mashed
- 1 tbsp lemon juice
- 1 celery stalk, diced
- 1 green onion, Sliced
- Salt and pepper,+

Instructions

1. Mash the avocado, lemon juice, and olive oil in a bowl.
2. If using, stir in Dijon mustard.
3. Add the green onion, celery, and tuna. Stir until incorporated.
4. As needed, add salt and pepper.
5. Serve with cucumber slices, on almond toast, or in lettuce wraps.

Notes

- ✓ Add chop-up pickles or capers for extra flavor.
- ✓ Keeps well in the fridge for up to 2 days.

Nutrition Info (Per Serving)

- Calories: 220
- Fat: 14g
- Carbs: 3g
- Fiber: 2g
- Sugar: 1g
- Protein: 20g

36. TURMERIC CHICKEN SKEWERS

Prep Time: 15 Mins

Cook Time: 15 Mins

Total Time: 30 Mins

Servings: 2

Ingredients

- 2 chicken breasts, cut into 1-inch cubes
- 2 tbsp olive oil
- 1 tbsp turmeric
- 1 tsp ground cumin
- 1 tsp paprika
- 1 tbsp lemon juice
- 2 cloves garlic, chop-up
- Sea salt and pepper,+
- Fresh cilantro for garnish

Instructions

1. In a bowl, mix the olive oil, lemon juice, garlic, paprika, turmeric, cumin, salt, and pepper.
2. After tossing the chicken cubes in the marinade, leave them for fifteen to twenty min.
3. Turn the heat up to medium-high on the grill or grill pan.
4. After skewering the chicken, grill it for 4 to 5 minutes on every side or until it is cooked.
5. Before serving, garnish with fresh cilantro.

Notes

- ✓ Serve these skewers with a side of grilled vegetables or over cauliflower rice.
- ✓ You can also bake the skewers in a 400°F (200°C) oven for 15–18 min.

Nutrition Info (Per Serving)

- Calories: 220
- Fat: 14g
- Carbs: 3g
- Fiber: 1g
- Sugar: 1g
- Protein: 24g

37. GRILLED PORTOBELLO MUSHROOMS

Prep Time: 5 Mins

Cook Time: 10 Mins

Total Time: 15 Mins

Servings: 2

Ingredients

- 4 large Portobello mushroom caps, stems removed
- 2 tbsp olive oil
- 1 tbsp balsamic vinegar
- 1 clove garlic, chop-up
- 1 tsp dried oregano
- Sea salt and black pepper,+

Instructions

1. Turn the heat up to medium-high on the grill or grill pan.
2. In a small bowl, mix the olive oil, balsamic vinegar, oregano, garlic, salt, and pepper.
3. Apply the olive oil mixture on both sides of the mushrooms.
4. Mushrooms should be juicy and soft after grilling for 4 to 5 min on every side.
5. Serve over a salad or as a side dish.

Notes

- ✓ These mushrooms can be served as a burger "bun" or paired with grilled chicken or steak.
- ✓ If you don't have a grill, roast them in the oven at 400°F (200°C) for 12 min.

Nutrition Info (Per Serving)

- Calories: 130
- Fat: 11g
- Carbs: 7g
- Fiber: 3g
- Sugar: 3g
- Protein: 3g

38. STUFFED BELL PEPPERS (WITH GROUND TURKEY)

Prep Time: 15 Mins

Cook Time: 30 Mins

Total Time: 45 Mins

Servings: 4

Ingredients

- 4 bell peppers, tops cut off and seeds removed
- ½lb ground turkey
- 1 tbsp olive oil
- 1 small onion, diced
- 2 cloves garlic, chop-up
- ½tsp dried oregano
- ½tsp paprika
- ¼ cup of tomato sauce (no sugar added)
- ¼ cup of chop-up fresh parsley
- Sea salt and pepper,+

Instructions

1. Turn the oven on to 375°F, or 190°C.
2. In a pan, heat the olive oil over medium heat. Sauté the garlic and onions for three min.
3. Season with salt, pepper, paprika, oregano, and ground turkey. Cook until browned.
4. Cook for a further two to three min after adding the tomato sauce. Take off the heat.
5. After stuffing the bell peppers with the turkey mixture, could you place them in a baking dish?
6. Bake the peppers for 25 to 30 min, covered with foil, or until soft.
7. Before serving, garnish with fresh parsley.

Notes

- ✓ Add cooked quinoa or cauliflower rice to the filling for extra bulk.
- ✓ For a dairy-free version, omit or add a dairy-free cheese alternative.

Nutrition Info (Per Serving)

- Calories: 230
- Fat: 12g
- Carbs: 10g
- Fiber: 3g
- Sugar: 5g
- Protein: 24g

39. GUT-HEALING COLLAGEN SOUP

Prep Time: 5 Mins

Cook Time: 15 Mins

Total Time: 20 Mins

Servings: 2

Ingredients

- 2 cups of chicken bone broth
- ¼ cup of collagen powder (unflavored)
- ½cup of chop-up carrots
- ½cup of chop-up celery
- ½cup of chop-up spinach
- 1 clove garlic, chop-up
- 1 tbsp apple cider vinegar
- Sea salt and pepper,+

Instructions

1. Heat the chicken bone broth in a saucepan over medium heat.
2. Simmer the spinach, carrots, celery, and garlic for ten minutes or until the vegetables are soft.
3. Add the collagen powder and stir until it dissolves.
4. Season with salt and pepper, then add apple cider vinegar.
5. Warm up and serve.

Notes

- ✓ Collagen powder is excellent for gut health and helps to heal the digestive system.
- ✓ You can add other veggies like zucchini or mushrooms for variety.

Nutrition Info (Per Serving)

- Calories: 180
- Fat: 6g
- Carbs: 6g
- Fiber: 2g
- Sugar: 2g
- Protein: 26g

40. LEMON AVOCADO TUNA SALAD

Total Time: 10 Mins

Servings: 2

Ingredients

- 1 can wild-caught tuna, drained
- 1 ripe avocado, diced
- 1 tbsp olive oil
- 1 tbsp lemon juice
- 1 tbsp chop-up fresh parsley
- 1 tbsp chop-up red onion (non-compulsory)
- Sea salt and black pepper,+

Instructions

1. In a bowl, combine the tuna, avocado, lemon juice, olive oil, parsley, and red onion (if using).
2. Toss gently to mix.
3. Add pepper and sea salt.
4. Serve right away or store in the refrigerator for later.

Notes

- ✓ This salad is a great option for meal prep, as it can be kept in the fridge for up to two days.
- ✓ You can serve it in lettuce wraps or on a bed of mixed greens.

Nutrition Info (Per Serving)

- Calories: 300
- Fat: 21g
- Carbs: 10g
- Fiber: 7g
- Sugar: 2g
- Protein: 22g

41. ROASTED CHICKEN THIGHS WITH BROCCOLI

Prep Time: 10 Mins

Cook Time: 40 Mins

Total Time: 50 Mins

Ingredients

- 4 bone-in, skin-on chicken thighs
- 2 tbsp olive oil
- 1 tsp garlic powder
- 1 tsp dried thyme
- 1 tsp paprika
- Sea salt and black pepper,+
- 4 cups of broccoli florets

Instructions

1. Turn the oven on to 400°F or 200°C.
2. In a small bowl, combine the olive oil, salt, pepper, paprika, garlic powder, and thyme.
3. Coat the chicken thighs with the mixture.
4. Place the chicken on a baking sheet and roast it for 35 to 40 minutes, or until the internal temperature reaches 165°F (75°C) and the skin is crispy.
5. Place broccoli florets on the same baking sheet and cook for the last 10 min.
6. To achieve consistent cooking, toss the broccoli once while roasting the chicken.
7. Serve the roasted broccoli beside the chicken thighs.

Notes

- ✓ For extra crispy skin, pat the chicken dry before seasoning.
- ✓ You can use other vegetables like carrots or cauliflower for variety.

Nutrition Info (Per Serving)

- Calories: 400
- Fat: 30g
- Carbs: 10g
- Fiber: 4g
- Sugar: 2g
- Protein: 28g

42. GRILLED LAMB CHOPS WITH MINT

Prep Time: 10 Mins

Cook Time: 8 Mins

Total Time: 18 Mins

Ingredients

- 4 lamb chops
- 2 tbsp olive oil
- 2 tbsp fresh mint, chop-up
- 1 tbsp lemon juice
- 2 cloves garlic, chop-up
- Sea salt and black pepper,+

Instructions

1. Turn the heat up to medium-high on the grill or grill pan.
2. In a small bowl, mix the lemon juice, garlic, olive oil, mint, salt, and pepper.
3. Let the lamb chops marinate for ten min after rubbing them with the mint mixture.
4. Lamb chops should be cooked to your preferred doneness, 4 min on every side.
5. Before serving, give the lamb chops five min to rest.

Notes

- ✓ Serve these lamb chops with roasted vegetables or a fresh salad for a complete meal.
- ✓ Lamb is a rich protein and healthy fat source, making this a great dinner option.

Nutrition Info (Per Serving)

- Calories: 350
- Fat: 25g
- Carbs: 2g
- Fiber: 1g
- Sugar: 1g
- Protein: 30g

43. CILANTRO LIME CAULIFLOWER RICE

Prep Time: 5 Min

Cook Time: 5 Min

Total Time: 10 Min

Servings: 4

Ingredients

- 1 medium cauliflower, finely grated or riced
- 1 tbsp olive oil
- 1 clove garlic, chop-up
- ¼ cup of fresh cilantro, chop up
- 1 tbsp lime juice
- Sea salt and pepper,+

Instructions

1. In a large skillet, heat the olive oil over medium heat.
2. Add the chop-up garlic and cook until fragrant, about 1 minute.
3. Cook, stirring periodically, for 4 to 5 min after adding the riced cauliflower.
4. Take off the heat and mix in the cilantro, lime juice, salt, and pepper.
5. Serve alongside your preferred protein.

Notes

- ✓ For extra flavor, add a pinch of cumin or chili flakes.
- ✓ This rice can be made and stored in the fridge for up to 3 days.

Nutrition Info (Per Serving)

- Calories: 45
- Fat: 3g
- Carbs: 5g
- Fiber: 2g
- Sugar: 2g
- Protein: 2g

44. BEEF AND CABBAGE STIR FRY

Prep Time: 10 Mins

Cook Time: 15 Mins

Total Time: 25 Mins

Servings: 4

Ingredients

- 1 lb ground beef
- 2 cup of shredded cabbage
- 1 tbsp olive oil

- 1 small onion, diced
- 2 cloves garlic, chop-up
- 2 tbsp coconut aminos (or tamari for a gluten-free option)
- 1 tsp ground ginger
- Sea salt and pepper,+

Instructions

1. In a large pan, heat the olive oil over medium-high heat.
2. Sauté the chop-up garlic and chop-up onion for two to three min or until they are tender.
3. Use a spoon to break up the ground beef once it has been added and cooked until browned.
4. Add the ginger, coconut aminos, shredded cabbage, salt, and pepper.
5. Cook, stirring occasionally, until the cabbage is soft, about 5 to 7 more min.
6. Enjoy it hot!

Notes

✓ You can swap ground beef for ground turkey or chicken if preferred.
✓ For added crunch, top with sesame seeds or chop up green onions.

Nutrition Info (Per Serving)

- Calories: 280
- Fat: 18g
- Carbs: 8g
- Fiber: 3g
- Sugar: 4g
- Protein: 24g

45. LEMON ROSEMARY BAKED SALMON

Prep Time: 5 Mins

Cook Time: 15 Mins

Total Time: 20 Mins

Servings: 2

Ingredients

- 2 salmon fillets (about 6 oz every)
- 2 tbsp olive oil
- 1 tbsp fresh rosemary, chop-up

- 1 lemon, thinly Sliced
- Sea salt and black pepper,+

Instructions

1. Set the oven's temperature to 400°F or 200°C.
2. Arrange the salmon fillets on a parchment paper-lined baking pan.
3. Season with salt and pepper, add rosemary and drizzle with olive oil.
4. Add slices of lemon on top.
5. Salmon should flake readily with a fork after 12 to 15 min of baking.
6. Serve alongside your preferred side dish.

Notes

✓ For extra flavor, you can add a drizzle of lemon juice right before serving.
✓ This dish pairs well with steamed vegetables or cauliflower rice.

Nutrition Info (Per Serving)

- Calories: 330
- Fat: 20g
- Carbs: 4g
- Fiber: 1g
- Sugar: 1g
- Protein: 30g

46. GARLIC BUTTER ZUCCHINI NOODLES

Prep Time: 5 Mins

Cook Time: 5 Mins

Total Time: 10 Mins

Servings: 2

Ingredients

- 2 medium zucchini, spiralized
- 2 tbsp butter (or ghee for dairy-free)
- 2 cloves garlic, chop-up
- 1 tbsp olive oil
- 1 tbsp fresh parsley, chop-up
- Sea salt and black pepper,+

Instructions

1. Melt the butter and olive oil over medium heat in a large skillet.
2. Add the chop-up garlic and cook until fragrant, about 1 minute.
3. Sauté the zucchini noodles for two to three min or until they are soft but still have some firmness.
4. Add fresh parsley and season with salt and pepper.
5. If preferred, top with more parsley and serve right away.

Notes

✓ You can add finely grated Parmesan or nutritional yeast for a cheesy flavor (non-compulsory).
✓ For a heartier dish, top with grilled chicken or shrimp.

Nutrition Info (Per Serving)

- Calories: 180
- Fat: 15g
- Carbs: 6g
- Fiber: 2g
- Sugar: 4g
- Protein: 2g

47. CAULIFLOWER AND COCONUT CURRY

Prep Time: 10 Mins

Cook Time: 20 Mins

Total Time: 30 Mins

Servings: 4

Ingredients

- 1 medium cauliflower, cut into florets
- 1 tbsp olive oil
- 1 small onion, diced
- 2 cloves garlic, chop-up
- 1 tbsp finely grated ginger
- 1 tbsp curry powder
- ½tsp turmeric
- 1 can (14 oz) coconut milk
- ½cup of vegetable broth

- 1 tbsp fresh cilantro, chop-up
- Sea salt and pepper,+

Instructions

1. In a large pan, heat the olive oil over medium heat.
2. Sauté the ginger, garlic, and Sliced onion for three to four min or until aromatic.
3. Cook for one minute after adding the curry powder, turmeric, and a touch of salt.
4. Add the vegetable broth, coconut milk, and cauliflower florets. Mix to blend.
5. Simmer until the cauliflower is soft, and the sauce has thickened 15 to 20 min.
6. Serve after adding some fresh cilantro as a garnish.

Notes

- ✓ You can add spinach or peas for extra vegetables.
- ✓ Serve with cauliflower rice for a complete low-carb meal.

Nutrition Info (Per Serving)

- Calories: 220
- Fat: 18g
- Carbs: 14g
- Fiber: 6g
- Sugar: 4g
- Protein: 4g

48. ROASTED BRUSSELS SPROUTS WITH TURKEY

Prep Time: 10 Mins

Cook Time: 30 Mins

Total Time: 40 Mins

Servings: 4

Ingredients

- 1 lb Brussels sprouts, halved
- 1 lb ground turkey
- 2 tbsp olive oil
- 1 tsp dried thyme
- 1 tsp garlic powder
- Sea salt and pepper,+

Instructions

1. Turn the oven on to 400°F or 200°C.
2. Add salt, pepper, garlic powder, thyme, and olive oil to the Brussels sprouts. Arrange them in an equal layer on a baking sheet.
3. Roast Brussels sprouts until golden and crispy, stirring for 20 to 25 min.
4. Heat a pan over medium heat while the sprouts roast. Using a spoon, break up the ground turkey while it cooks until browned.
5. Add the roasted Brussels sprouts and season the turkey with salt and pepper.
6. Warm up and serve.

Notes

✓ For extra flavor, add a drizzle of balsamic vinegar to the Brussels sprouts before roasting.
✓ While cooking, you can also add a handful of chopped onions to the turkey.

Nutrition Info (Per Serving)

- Calories: 300
- Fat: 18g
- Carbs: 10g
- Fiber: 4g
- Sugar: 3g
- Protein: 28g

49. SPAGHETTI SQUASH PAD THAI

Prep Time: 10 Mins

Cook Time: 25 Mins

Total Time: 35 Mins

Servings: 2

Ingredients

- 1 medium spaghetti squash
- 2 tbsp coconut oil
- ¼ cup of coconut aminos (or tamari)
- 1 tbsp lime juice
- 2 eggs, scrambled
- ½cup of shredded carrots
- ¼ cup of chop-up green onions

- ¼ cup of chop-up cilantro
- 1 tbsp chop-up peanuts (non-compulsory)
- Sea salt and pepper,+

Instructions

1. Turn the oven on to 400°F or 200°C.
2. Place spaghetti squash face down on a baking sheet after halving it and removing the seeds.
3. Roast until soft, about 25 min. Shred the meat into spaghetti-like pieces using a fork.
4. In a large pan, heat the coconut oil over medium heat. Add the lime juice and coconut aminos.
5. After adding the scrambled eggs and cooking until set, toss the shredded spaghetti squash, carrots, green onions, and cilantro.
6. Mix thoroughly, and if you'd like, top with peanuts.

Notes

✓ You can add shrimp or chicken for extra protein.
✓ This dish can be served warm or cold as a salad.

Nutrition Info (Per Serving)

- Calories: 220
- Fat: 15g
- Carbs: 18g
- Fiber: 5g
- Sugar: 5g
- Protein: 8g

50. BALSAMIC GRILLED VEGETABLES

Prep Time: 10 Mins

Cook Time: 15 Mins

Total Time: 25 Mins

Servings: 4

Ingredients

- 2 zucchinis, Sliced
- 1 bell pepper, cut into strips
- 1 red onion, cut into wedges

- 1 cup of cherry tomatoes, halved
- 3 tbsp balsamic vinegar
- 2 tbsp olive oil
- 1 tsp dried oregano
- Sea salt and pepper,+

Instructions

1. Turn the heat up to medium-high on the grill or grill pan.
2. Balsamic vinegar, olive oil, oregano, salt, and pepper should all be mixed in a bowl.
3. Make sure the veggies are well covered by tossing them in the balsamic mixture.
4. Vegetables should be soft and browned on the grill after 10 to 15 min, flipping periodically.
5. If preferred, top with more balsamic drizzle and serve warm.

Notes

✓ You can also roast these vegetables in the oven at 400°F (200°C) for 20 min.
✓ It is excellent as a side dish or tossed into a salad.

Nutrition Info (Per Serving)

- Calories: 120
- Fat: 9g
- Carbs: 15g
- Fiber: 6g
- Sugar: 6g
- Protein: 2g

51. KETO CHICKEN ALFREDO (WITH CAULIFLOWER SAUCE)

Prep Time: 10 Mins

Cook Time: 25 Mins

Total Time: 35 Mins

Servings: 4

Ingredients

- 4 boneless, skinless chicken breasts
- 1 tbsp olive oil
- 1 small head cauliflower, chop-up

- 2 cloves garlic, chop-up
- 1 cup of unsweetened almond milk
- ¼ cup of finely grated Parmesan cheese
- 1 tbsp nutritional yeast (non-compulsory)
- Sea salt and pepper,+
- Fresh parsley, chop-up (for garnish)

Instructions

1. Turn the heat up to medium-high on the grill or grill pan.
2. Balsamic vinegar, olive oil, oregano, salt, and pepper should all be mixed in a bowl.
3. Make sure the veggies are well covered by tossing them in the balsamic mixture.
4. Vegetables should be soft and browned on the grill after 10 to 15 min, flipping periodically.
5. If preferred, top with more balsamic drizzle and serve warm.In a pan, heat the olive oil over medium heat. Add salt and pepper to the chicken breasts and cook for 6 to 7 minutes on every side or until cooked through and golden. Remove and place aside from the skillet.
6. Add the chop-up cauliflower and garlic to the same skillet. Sauté for two to three min.
7. After adding the almond milk, bring to a simmer. Cover and simmer for approximately 10 minutes or until the cauliflower is soft.
8. In a food processor or blender, mix the cauliflower and cooking liquid. Blend until smooth. If using, stir in nutritional yeast and Parmesan cheese. Adjust the seasoning with salt and pepper.
9. After cutting the chicken, serve it with the Alfredo sauce for cauliflower. Add some fresh parsley as a garnish.

Notes

✓ You can serve this with zucchini noodles or steamed broccoli for added vegetables.
✓ Add a splash of heavy cream to the cauliflower sauce for a creamier texture.

Nutrition Info (Per Serving)

- Calories: 300
- Fat: 15g
- Carbs: 8g
- Fiber: 3g
- Sugar: 3g
- Protein: 34g

52. CABBAGE AND MUSHROOM STIR FRY

Prep Time: 5 Mins

Cook Time: 10 Mins

Total Time: 15 Mins

Servings: 4

Ingredients

- 2 cup of shredded cabbage
- 1 cup of mushrooms, Sliced
- 2 tbsp coconut oil
- 1 tbsp coconut aminos (or tamari)
- ½tsp ground ginger
- 1 tbsp sesame seeds (non-compulsory)
- Sea salt and pepper,+

Instructions

1. In a large pan, heat the coconut oil over medium heat.
2. Cook the Sliced mushrooms for three to four minutes or until tender.
3. Stir-fry the shredded cabbage for five to seven minutes or until it is soft.
4. Add ginger, salt, pepper, and coconut aminos. Cook for a further minute.
5. If preferred, garnish with sesame seeds and serve hot.

Notes

- ✓ To make this a complete meal, you can add protein, like shrimp or chicken.
- ✓ For extra flavor, top with chop-up green onions or a drizzle of sriracha (if tolerated).

Nutrition Info (Per Serving)

- Calories: 150
- Fat: 10g
- Carbs: 12g
- Fiber: 5g
- Sugar: 5g
- Protein: 3g

53. COCONUT CRUSTED COD

Prep Time: 10 Mins

Cook Time: 15 Mins

Total Time: 25 Mins

Servings: 4

Ingredients

- 4 cod fillets (about 6 oz every)
- ½cup of shredded unsweetened coconut
- ¼ cup of almond flour
- 1 egg, beaten
- 1 tbsp coconut oil
- 1 tsp garlic powder
- 1 tsp paprika
- Sea salt and pepper,+

Instructions

1. Set the oven's temperature to 400°F or 200°C. Put parchment paper on a baking pan.
2. Add the shredded coconut, almond flour, paprika, garlic powder, salt, and pepper to a shallow dish.
3. Coat every fish fillet with the coconut mixture after dipping it in the beaten egg.
4. In a pan, heat the coconut oil over medium heat. Add the cod fillets and fry until golden and crispy, 2 to 3 min per side when heated.
5. Place the fillets on the baking pan and bake for 8 to 10 minutes or until they are flaky and cooked through.
6. Serve with a lemon squeeze.

Notes

- ✓ Cod can be substituted with other white fish like tilapia or haddock.
- ✓ Pair with a sautéed spinach or a fresh salad for a complete meal.

Nutrition Info (Per Serving)

- Calories: 280
- Fat: 18g
- Carbs: 6g
- Fiber: 3g
- Sugar: 2g
- Protein: 26g

54. GRILLED EGGPLANT WITH TAHINI SAUCE

Prep Time: 10 Mins

Cook Time: 15 Mins

Total Time: 25 Mins

Servings: 4

Ingredients

- 2 medium eggplants, Sliced into rounds
- 2 tbsp olive oil
- ¼ tsp ground cumin
- Sea salt and pepper,+
- ¼ cup of tahini
- 1 tbsp lemon juice
- 1 tbsp water (to thin sauce)
- 1 clove garlic, chop-up
- Fresh parsley, chop-up (for garnish)

Instructions

1. Turn the heat up to medium-high on the grill or grill pan.
2. Sprinkle the eggplant slices with salt, pepper, and cumin after brushing them with olive oil.
3. The eggplant should be soft and have grill marks on every side after 3–4 min.
4. Mix the tahini, water, lemon juice, and garlic in a small bowl and whisk until smooth.
5. Garnish the grilled eggplant slices with fresh parsley and drizzle them with the tahini sauce.

Notes

- ✓ You can also roast the eggplant in the oven at 400°F (200°C) for 20–25 min.
- ✓ This dish pairs well with grilled chicken or a fresh salad.

Nutrition Info (Per Serving)

- Calories: 200
- Fat: 18g
- Carbs: 10g
- Fiber: 5g
- Sugar: 4g

- Protein: 4g

55. TURMERIC BEEF MEATBALLS

Prep Time: 10 Mins

Cook Time: 20 Mins

Total Time: 30 Mins

Servings: 4

Ingredients

- 1 lb ground beef
- 1 egg
- 2 tbsp almond flour
- 1 tbsp turmeric powder
- 1 tsp garlic powder
- 1 tsp ground cumin
- ½tsp salt
- ¼ tsp black pepper
- 2 tbsp olive oil (for frying)

Instructions

1. Turn the oven on to 375°F, or 190°C.
2. Combine the ground beef, egg, almond flour, cumin, turmeric, garlic powder, salt, and pepper in a mixing bowl and stir until well blended.
3. On a baking sheet, form the mixture into 1-inch meatballs.
4. In a pan, heat the olive oil over medium heat. Brown the meatballs for two to three minutes on each side.
5. The browned meatballs should be cooked after 12 to 15 minutes of baking.
6. Serve hot over cauliflower rice or over steamed veggies.

Notes

- ✓ You can add fresh chop-up parsley or cilantro for added freshness.
- ✓ These meatballs freeze well and can be stored in an airtight container for up to 3 months.

Nutrition Info (Per Serving)

- Calories: 320
- Fat: 23g
- Carbs: 4g

- Fiber: 1g
- Sugar: 1g
- Protein: 28g

56. CHICKEN AND KALE STEW

Prep Time: 10 Mins

Cook Time: 40 Mins

Total Time: 50 Mins

Servings: 4

Ingredients

- 2 boneless, skinless chicken breasts, diced
- 4 cups of chicken broth (preferably homemade or low-sodium)
- 2 cups of kale, chop up
- 1 small onion, diced
- 2 cloves garlic, chop-up
- 2 carrots, Sliced
- 1 celery stalk, chop-up
- 1 tsp dried thyme
- 1 tbsp olive oil
- Sea salt and pepper,+

Instructions

1. In a large saucepan, heat the olive oil over medium heat. Cook the chopped onion and garlic for approximately two minutes or until tender.
2. Cook the chop-up chicken breasts in the saucepan for five to seven min or until they are browned.
3. Add the kale, carrots, celery, salt, pepper, and thyme.
4. Add the chicken broth, boil, and cook until the veggies are soft for about 30 minutes.
5. Serve hot, adjusting the spice as necessary.

Notes

- ✓ For more variety, you can add vegetables, such as zucchini or squash.
- ✓ This stew can be stored in the refrigerator for up to 3 days or frozen for up to 3 months.

Nutrition Info (Per Serving)

- Calories: 250
- Fat: 12g
- Carbs: 10g
- Fiber: 3g
- Sugar: 4g
- Protein: 26g

57. MISO GINGER SOUP (WITH ZUCCHINI NOODLES)

Prep Time: 5 Mins

Cook Time: 10 Mins

Total Time: 15 Mins

Servings: 2

Ingredients

- 4 cups of vegetable broth
- 2 tbsp miso paste (look for a sugar-free version)
- 1-inch piece of fresh ginger, finely grated
- 1 medium zucchini, spiralized into noodles
- 1 tbsp coconut aminos (or tamari for gluten-free)
- ½cup of mushrooms, Sliced
- 1 green onion, chop up (for garnish)
- Sea salt and pepper,+

Instructions

1. Put the coconut aminos, finely grated ginger, miso paste, and vegetable broth in a big saucepan. Please stir it to dissolve the miso paste.
2. Over medium heat, bring the broth to a boil and cook for five min.
3. Add the cut mushrooms and zucchini noodles to the broth. Cook until the zucchini is soft, about 2 to 3 more minutes.
4. As needed, add salt and pepper.
5. Serve hot, garnished with chop-up green onion.

Notes

- ✓ This soup can be made over time and stored in the fridge for up to 3 days.
- ✓ You can add tofu or shrimp for added protein.

Nutrition Info (Per Serving)

- Calories: 120
- Fat: 5g
- Carbs: 12g
- Fiber: 4g
- Sugar: 5g
- Protein: 4g

58. PALEO SHEPHERD'S PIE (CAULIFLOWER MASH)

Prep Time: 15 Mins

Cook Time: 30 Mins

Total Time: 45 Mins

Servings: 4

Ingredients

- 1 lb ground beef (or lamb)
- 1 small onion, diced
- 2 cloves garlic, chop-up
- 2 carrots, diced
- ½cup of peas (non-compulsory)
- 2 tbsp tomato paste
- 1 cup of beef broth
- 1 head cauliflower, chop-up
- 2 tbsp olive oil (for cauliflower mash)
- ¼ cup of coconut milk
- Sea salt and pepper,+

Instructions

1. Set the oven's temperature to 400°F or 200°C.
2. Break the ground beef with a spoon and sauté it over medium heat in a large pan until it is browned.
3. Cook the chopped carrots, onion, and garlic in the skillet for five minutes or until tender.
4. Add the beef broth, tomato paste, and peas (if using). Simmer until the mixture thickens, 5 to 7 minutes. Season with salt and pepper.

5. In the meantime, steam the cauliflower for ten minutes or until it is soft. Add the coconut milk and olive oil to the cauliflower and mash until smooth—season with salt and pepper.
6. The beef mixture should be moved to a baking dish. Evenly distribute the mashed cauliflower on top.
7. Bake for 10 to 15 min or until golden and crispy on top.
8. Warm up and serve.

Notes

✓ You can substitute ground turkey or chicken for beef for a lighter version.
✓ If you prefer, add some fresh herbs like rosemary or thyme to the cauliflower mash.

Nutrition Info (Per Serving)

- Calories: 350
- Fat: 22g
- Carbs: 18g
- Fiber: 6g
- Sugar: 7g
- Protein: 24g

59. LMOND CRUSTED CHICKEN TENDERS

Prep Time: 10 Mins

Cook Time: 20 Mins

Total Time: 30 Mins

Servings: 4

Ingredients

- 1 lb chicken tenders
- 1 cup of almond flour
- 1 tsp garlic powder
- 1 tsp paprika
- ½tsp sea salt
- ¼ tsp black pepper
- 2 eggs, beaten
- 2 tbsp olive oil (for cooking)

Instructions

1. Put parchment paper on a baking pan and preheat the oven to 400°F (200°C).
2. Whisk the eggs in a bowl. Mix the almond flour, paprika, garlic powder, salt, and pepper in a separate bowl.
3. Coat every chicken tender with the almond flour mixture after dipping it in the egg.
4. On the baking sheet, arrange the coated tenders. Lightly drizzle with olive oil.
5. Bake for 18 to 20 min, turning halfway through, until cooked through and brown.

Notes

✓ You can also air fry these at 375°F for 12–15 min for a crispier texture.
✓ Delicious with a sugar-free mustard dip.

Nutrition Info (Per Serving)

- Calories: 320
- Fat: 20g
- Carbs: 6g
- Fiber: 2g
- Sugar: 1g
- Protein: 30g

60. GARLIC HERB BAKED COD

Prep Time: 5 Mins

Cook Time: 15 Mins

Total Time: 20 Mins

Servings: 2

Ingredients

- 2 cod fillets
- 2 tbsp olive oil
- 2 cloves garlic, chop-up
- 1 tbsp fresh parsley, chop-up
- 1 tbsp lemon juice
- Salt and pepper,+

Instructions

1. Turn the oven on to 400°F or 200°C. Cod fillets should be put on a baking dish.

2. In a small bowl, combine the lemon juice, parsley, garlic, olive oil, salt, and pepper.
3. Evenly spoon the mixture over the fish.
4. The fish should flake readily with a fork after 12 to 15 min of baking.

Notes

✓ Serve with steamed vegetables or cauliflower rice for a complete meal.
✓ Fresh herbs like thyme or dill also pair beautifully with cod.

Nutrition Info (Per Serving

+ Calories: 230
+ Fat: 14g
+ Carbs: 2g
+ Fiber: 0g
+ Sugar: 0g
+ Protein: 22g

61. CUCUMBER AVOCADO BITES

Total Time: 10 Mins

Servings: 4

Ingredients

- 1 large cucumber, Sliced into rounds
- 1 ripe avocado
- 1 tbsp lemon juice
- 1 tbsp olive oil
- 1 garlic clove, chop-up
- Sea salt and pepper,+
- Fresh dill or parsley for garnish

Instructions

1. Mash the avocado, lemon juice, olive oil, and chopped garlic in a small bowl.
2. Add salt and pepper for seasoning.
3. Place a spoonful of the avocado mixture on top of every piece of cucumber.
4. Before serving, garnish with parsley or fresh dill.

Notes

✓ You can sprinkle a few hemp seeds on top for added texture and protein.
✓ Serve immediately for the best flavor and texture.

Nutrition Info (Per Serving

- Calories: 120
- Fat: 10g
- Carbs: 7g
- Fiber: 3g
- Sugar: 2g
- Protein: 2g

62. COCONUT CHIPS (HOMEMADE)

Prep Time: 5 Mins

Cook Time: 15 Mins

Total Time: 20 Min

Servings: 4

Ingredients

- 1 cup of unsweetened shredded coconut
- 1 tbsp coconut oil
- ¼ tsp sea salt
- ¼ tsp cinnamon (non-compulsory)

Instructions

1. Set the oven's temperature to 175°C (350°F). Put parchment paper on a baking pan.
2. Shredded coconut, melted coconut oil, salt, and cinnamon (if used) should all be mixed in a mixing bowl.
3. On the baking sheet that has been prepared, evenly distribute the coconut mixture.
4. To guarantee even browning, stir every five minutes while baking for ten to fifteen minutes. Because coconut may burn fast, pay cautious attention.
5. Please remove it from the oven and let it cool once it is brown and crispy.

Notes

- ✓ Store in an airtight container for up to 1 week.
- ✓ You can adjust the flavor by adding a bit of vanilla extract or a sprinkle of stevia if you prefer a sweeter taste.

Nutrition Info (Per Serving)

- Calories: 180
- Fat: 18g
- Carbs: 6g
- Fiber: 4g
- Sugar: 1g
- Protein: 2g

63. KALE CHIPS (NO SUGAR)

Prep Time: 10 Mins

Cook Time: 15-20 Mins

Total Time: 25-30 Mins

Servings: 4

Ingredients

- 1 bunch of kale, washed and dried
- 1 tbsp olive oil
- ½tsp sea salt
- ¼ tsp garlic powder (non-compulsory)
- ¼ tsp smoked paprika (non-compulsory)

Instructions

1. Set the oven's temperature to 175°C (350°F). Put parchment paper on a baking pan.
2. Tear the kale leaves into bite-sized pieces after removing them from the stems.
3. Mix the kale, salt, olive oil, and other ingredients in a big bowl.
4. On the baking sheet, equally distribute the kale, ensuring that the leaves are in a single layer.
5. To avoid burning, check the oven every five minutes while baking for 15 to 20 minutes. When crispy, remove it from the oven and allow it to cool.

Notes

- ✓ Kale chips are best served immediately after cooling, as they can lose their crispiness over time.
- ✓ Store in an airtight container for up to 2-3 days.

Nutrition Info (Per Serving)

- Calories: 80
- Fat: 7g

- Carbs: 6g
- Fiber: 2g
- Sugar: 1g
- Protein: 2g

64. ALMOND BUTTER CELERY STICKS

Total Time: 5 Mins

Servings: 4

Ingredients

- 4 celery stalks, washed and cut into 3-inch pieces
- ¼ cup of almond butter (unsweetened)
- 1 tbsp chia seeds (non-compulsory, for extra fiber)
- Sea salt,+

Instructions

1. Cut the celery into 3-inch pieces after washing it.
2. Drizzle every celery stick with a large dollop of almond butter.
3. Add a touch of sea salt and some chia seeds.
4. Serve right away as an appetizer or snack.

Notes

- ✓ You can substitute almond butter with sunflower seed butter if you prefer a nut-free version.
- ✓ If you're making this snack ahead of time, store the almond butter-filled celery sticks in the fridge for up to 1 day.

Nutrition Info (Per Serving)

- Calories: 180
- Fat: 16g
- Carbs: 8g
- Fiber: 5g
- Sugar: 2g
- Protein: 6g

65. COCONUT FAT BOMBS

Prep Time: 10 Mins

Total Time: 10 min + 1-2 hrs chill time

Servings: 12

Ingredients

- ½cup of coconut oil, melted
- ¼ cup of unsweetened shredded coconut
- 2 tbsp almond butter or coconut butter
- 1 tbsp chia seeds (non-compulsory)
- ½tsp vanilla extract
- ¼ tsp sea salt
- 2 tbsp stevia or erythritol (non-compulsory, for sweetness)

Instructions

1. Melted coconut oil, shredded coconut, almond butter, chia seeds, sea salt, and vanilla essence should all be mixed in a mixing dish.
2. If desired, add erythritol or stevia for sweetness.
3. Put the mixture in the freezer after pouring it into silicone molds or an ice cube tray.
4. Freeze until solid, about 1 to 2 hours. When the fat bombs are set, remove them from the molds.
5. Keep in the refrigerator for up to two weeks or in the freezer for up to three months in an airtight container.

Notes

- ✓ You can substitute almond butter with peanut butter if you prefer.
- ✓ For added flavor, you can mix in some cocoa powder or cinnamon.

Nutrition Info (Per Serving)

- Calories: 150
- Fat: 14g
- Carbs: 4g
- Fiber: 3g
- Sugar: 1g
- Protein: 2g

66. GUACAMOLE WITH VEGGIE STICKS

Total Time: 10 Mins

Servings: 4

Ingredients

- 2 ripe avocados, peeled and pitted
- ¼ cup of red onion, lightly chop up
- 1 small tomato, diced
- 1 tbsp fresh lime juice
- 1 tsp garlic powder
- ¼ tsp sea salt
- ¼ tsp black pepper
- Veggie sticks (carrots, cucumber, bell peppers) for dipping

Instructions

1. Using a fork, mash the avocados in a medium bowl until they are smooth but still have some chunks.
2. Add the lime juice, chop-up onion, tomato, salt, pepper, and garlic powder. Stir well.
3. Add lime juice, salt, or pepper to taste and adjust the seasoning.
4. Serve right away and provide fresh vegetable sticks for dipping.

Notes

- ✓ You can also add chop-up cilantro or a dash of cumin for extra flavor.
- ✓ This guacamole can be stored in the fridge for up to 1 day, but it's best served fresh.

Nutrition Info (Per Serving)

- Calories: 180
- Fat: 15g
- Carbs: 10g
- Fiber: 7g
- Sugar: 2g
- Protein: 2g

67. ROASTED SEAWEED SNACKS

Prep Time: 5 Mins

Cook Time: 5-7 Mins

Total Time: 10-12 Mins

Servings: 4

Ingredients

- 1 sheet nori seaweed (found in Asian grocery stores)
- 1 tsp sesame oil or olive oil
- ¼ tsp sea salt
- ¼ tsp garlic powder (non-compulsory)

Instructions

1. Set the oven's temperature to 175°C (350°F). Put parchment paper on a baking pan.
2. Apply sesame or olive oil to the nori sheet's two sides.
3. If used, sprinkle with garlic powder and sea salt.
4. Using scissors, cut the nori sheet into smaller squares or strips.
5. Arrange the pieces in a single layer on the baking sheet and bake for five to seven min or until they are crispy.
6. Before serving, let it cool.

Notes

- ✓ You can store roasted seaweed snacks in an airtight container for up to 1 week.
- ✓ These make a great low-carb snack or a topping for salads.

Nutrition Info (Per Serving)

- Calories: 35
- Fat: 2g
- Carbs: 4g
- Fiber: 1g
- Sugar: 0g
- Protein: 1g

68. TURMERIC ROASTED ALMONDS

Prep Time: 5 Mins

Cook Time: 15 Mins

Total Time: 20 Mins

Servings: 4

Ingredients

- 1 cup of raw almonds
- 1 tbsp olive oil or coconut oil

- 1 tsp turmeric powder
- ½tsp cumin powder
- ¼ tsp sea salt
- ¼ tsp black pepper

Instructions

1. Set the oven's temperature to 175°C (350°F). Put parchment paper on a baking pan.
2. In a small bowl, mix the almonds, cumin, turmeric powder, olive oil, salt, and pepper.
3. Arrange the seasoned almonds on the baking sheet in a single layer.
4. Roast until the almonds are aromatic and brown, stirring halfway through, 10 to 15 min.
5. Before serving, take it out of the oven and allow it to cool.

Notes

- ✓ Store the roasted almonds in an airtight container for up to 2 weeks.
- ✓ You can adjust the seasoning by adding a pinch of chili powder for a spicier kick.

Nutrition Info (Per Serving)

- Calories: 180
- Fat: 15g
- Carbs: 6g
- Fiber: 3g
- Sugar: 1g
- Protein: 6g

69. AVOCADO CUCUMBER SALAD

Total Time: 10 Mins

Servings: 4

Ingredients

- 1 large cucumber, Sliced
- 1 ripe avocado, diced
- 1 tbsp fresh lemon juice
- 1 tbsp olive oil
- ¼ tsp sea salt
- ¼ tsp black pepper
- Fresh herbs (parsley or dill) for garnish (non-compulsory)

Instructions

1. Cut the avocado into small pieces and slice the cucumber.
2. Put the avocado and cucumber in a big bowl.
3. Season with salt and pepper after drizzling with lemon juice and olive oil.
4. Add fresh herbs as a garnish after gently tossing to mix.
5. You may serve it immediately or chill it for up to an hr.

Notes

✓ This salad can be made in advance, but it's best served fresh to prevent the avocado from browning.
✓ For added flavor, sprinkle some feta cheese (if not dairy-free) or a few crushed nuts.

Nutrition Info (Per Serving)

- Calories: 180
- Fat: 15g
- Carbs: 12g
- Fiber: 7g
- Sugar: 3g
- Protein: 3g

70. BONE BROTH SIPPING CUP OF

Prep Time: 5 Mins

Cook Time: 5 Mins

Total Time: 10 Mins

Servings: 4

Ingredients

- 2 cups of bone broth (preferably homemade or organic)
- 1 tsp turmeric powder
- ½tsp black pepper
- 1 tbsp apple cider vinegar (non-compulsory, for tang)
- Fresh herbs (parsley, thyme, or rosemary) for garnish

Instructions

1. Transfer the bone broth to a saucepan and bring it to a warm temperature over medium heat.
2. Add the apple cider vinegar (if using), black pepper, and turmeric and stir.

3. To drink, transfer the soup into little cups.
4. Serve right away after garnishing with fresh herbs.

Notes

- ✓ This can be made with any bone broth—chicken, beef, or turkey.
- ✓ You can drink it as a savory snack or a base for other dishes.
- ✓ Adjust the seasoning or add a dash of cayenne for heat if you prefer a stronger flavor.

Nutrition Info (Per Serving)

- Calories: 40
- Fat: 1g
- Carbs: 2g
- Protein: 8g

71. FERMENTED VEGGIES (SUGAR-FREE)

Prep Time: 15 Mins

Total Time: 3-5 Days

Servings: 6

Ingredients

- 1 medium cucumber, Sliced
- 2 medium carrots, peeled and Sliced
- ½small head of cauliflower broken into florets
- 1 tbsp sea salt
- 2 cups of filtered water
- 1 garlic clove, smashed (non-compulsory)
- 1 tsp mustard seeds (non-compulsory)

Instructions

1. Mix the mustard seeds, cauliflower, carrots, cucumber, and garlic in a big glass jar.
2. Make a brine by dissolving the sea salt in filtered water in a different basin.
3. Cover the veggies with the brine, ensuring they are well submerged. If necessary, use a weight to hold them down.
4. Depending on how tangy you want your veggies, seal the jar and let it sit at room temperature for three to five days.
5. Please keep it in the fridge for up to two weeks after fermentation.

Notes

- ✓ Fermentation times can vary depending on the temperature of your kitchen. The warmer it is, the quicker the fermentation.
- ✓ Use this mixture as a snack, salad topper, or side dish.
- ✓ You can experiment with other vegetables like bell peppers or radishes.

Nutrition Info (Per Serving)

- ✦ Calories: 15
- ✦ Fat: 0g
- ✦ Carbs: 4g
- ✦ Fiber: 2g
- ✦ Sugar: 1g
- ✦ Protein: 1g

72. STUFFED AVOCADOS

Total Time: 10 Mins

Servings: 4

Ingredients

- 2 ripe avocados, halved and pitted
- ¼ cup of diced cucumber
- ¼ cup of diced tomato
- 1 tbsp lime juice
- 1 tbsp chop-up cilantro
- Sea salt and pepper+
- 1 tbsp olive oil (non-compulsory)

Instructions

1. Halve the avocados and scoop out the pits.
2. Mix the cucumber, tomato, cilantro, lime juice, salt, and pepper in a small bowl.
3. Place the mixture in the middle of every side of an avocado.
4. Garnish with more cilantro and drizzle with olive oil if you like.
5. Serve right away.

Notes

- ✓ You can top the stuffed avocados with grilled chicken or shrimp for added protein.
- ✓ These can be made and stored in the fridge for up to 1 day before serving.

✓ For more flavor, add other ingredients like red onion, jalapeño, or crumbled feta cheese.

Nutrition Info (Per Serving)

- Calories: 200
- Fat: 18g
- Carbs: 10g
- Fiber: 7g
- Sugar: 2g
- Protein: 3g

73. SPICED PUMPKIN SEEDS

Prep Time: 5 Mins

Cook Time: 15 Mins

Total Time: 20 Mins

Servings: 4

Ingredients

- 1 cup of pumpkin seeds (raw or roasted)
- 1 tbsp olive oil
- ½tsp paprika
- ½tsp cumin
- ¼ tsp turmeric
- ¼ tsp sea salt
- Pinch of black pepper

Instructions

1. Set the oven's temperature to 175°C (350°F). Put parchment paper on a baking pan.
2. Put the olive oil, turmeric, cumin, paprika, salt, and pepper in a small bowl.
3. Coat the pumpkin seeds thoroughly by tossing them in the spiced oil mixture.
4. Arrange the seeds on the baking sheet in a single layer.
5. Roast until the seeds are brown and crispy, 12 to 15 min, stirring once in between.
6. Before serving, allow to cool.

Notes

- ✓ You can store these spiced pumpkin seeds in an airtight container for up to 1 week.
- ✓ You can adjust the spices to your liking. For example, you can add a little cayenne for heat or cinnamon for a sweeter flavor.

Nutrition Info (Per Serving)

- Calories: 180
- Fat: 14g
- Carbs: 6g
- Fiber: 2g
- Sugar: 1g
- Protein: 10g

74. LEMON TAHINI DRESSING OVER CABBAGE

Total Time: 5 Mins

Servings: 4

Ingredients

- ¼ cup of tahini
- 2 tbsp fresh lemon juice
- 1 tbsp olive oil
- 1 tbsp water (to thin if necessary)
- ½tsp garlic powder
- ¼ tsp sea salt
- ¼ tsp black pepper
- 4 cups of shredded cabbage (green or purple)

Instructions

1. Mix the tahini, lemon juice, water, olive oil, garlic powder, salt, and pepper in a small bowl and whisk until smooth and creamy.
2. Toss the shredded cabbage with the tahini dressing in a large bowl until it's uniformly covered.
3. You may serve it immediately or chill it for up to an hr.

Notes

- ✓ This dressing also works as a drizzle for roasted vegetables or a dip for raw veggie sticks.

- ✓ If you prefer a thinner consistency, add more water or lemon juice until you reach your desired texture.

Nutrition Info (Per Serving)

- Calories: 120
- Fat: 10g
- Carbs: 6g
- Fiber: 3g
- Sugar: 3g
- Protein: 3g

75. BEET AND CABBAGE SLAW

Total Time: 10 Mins

Servings: 4

Ingredients

- 1 medium beet, peeled and finely grated
- 2 cups of shredded cabbage (green or purple)
- 1 tbsp apple cider vinegar
- 1 tbsp olive oil
- 1 tsp honey (non-compulsory)
- ¼ tsp sea salt
- ¼ tsp black pepper
- 1 tbsp chop-up fresh parsley (non-compulsory)

Instructions

1. Put the shredded cabbage and finely grated beet in a big basin.
2. Mix the apple cider vinegar, olive oil, honey (if using), salt, and pepper in a small bowl and whisk to mix.
3. Drizzle the beet and cabbage mixture with the dressing and toss to coat evenly.
4. Serve right away after adding some fresh parsley as a garnish.

Notes

- ✓ This slaw can be stored in the refrigerator for up to 2 days.
- ✓ You can adjust the sweetness by adding more honey if desired.
- ✓ For extra crunch, you can add sunflower seeds or pumpkin seeds.

Nutrition Info (Per Serving)

- Calories: 80

- Fat: 5g
- Carbs: 12g
- Fiber: 5g
- Sugar: 6g
- Protein: 2g

76. GINGER GARLIC BROCCOLI

Prep Time: 5 Mins

Cook Time: 5-7 Mins

Total Time: 10-12 Mins

Servings: 4

Ingredients

- 4 cups of broccoli florets
- 1 tbsp olive oil
- 2 cloves garlic, chop-up
- 1 tsp fresh ginger, finely grated
- 1 tbsp coconut aminos (or soy sauce)
- ¼ tsp sea salt
- ¼ tsp black pepper

Instructions

1. After two to three minutes of steaming or blanching in hot water, the broccoli florets should be brilliant green and crisp tender.
2. Heat the olive oil in a large pan over medium heat. Saut the finely grated ginger and chop uchoppedp garlic for one to twominutes,n or until fragrant.
3. Coat the cooked broccoli with the ginger and garlic by tossing it in the pan.
4. Add salt and pepper, drizzle with coconut aminos, and toss one more to mix.
5. Serve right away.

Notes

✓ You can add a pinch of red pepper flakes to the skillet for a bit of heat.
✓ This dish can also be served with grilled chicken or fish for a complete meal.

Nutrition Info (Per Serving)

- Calories: 90
- Fat: 7g
- Carbs: 9g

- Fiber: 4g
- Sugar: 2g
- Protein: 3g

77. BAKED CAULIFLOWER BITES

Prep Time: 10 Mins

Cook Time: 20 Mins

Total Time: 30 Mins

Servings: 4

Ingredients

- 1 medium head of cauliflower, cut into florets
- 2 tbsp olive oil
- 1 tsp garlic powder
- ½tsp paprika
- ¼ tsp sea salt
- ¼ tsp black pepper
- 1 tbsp fresh parsley, chop-up (non-compulsory)

Instructions

1. Put parchment paper on a baking pan and preheat the oven to 400°F (200°C).
2. Toss the cauliflower florets in a big basin with salt, pepper, paprika, garlic powder, and olive oil until they are uniformly covered.
3. Arrange the cauliflower florets on the prepared baking sheet in a single layer.
4. Bake the cauliflower for 20 min, turning halfway through, until the edges are brown and crispy.
5. Before serving, please remove it from the oven and top it with chop-up parsley.

Notes

- ✓ For extra crispiness, you can broil the cauliflower bites for the last 2 min of cooking.
- ✓ These make a great side dish or snack and pair well with a dipping sauce like tahini or coconut yogurt.

Nutrition Info (Per Serving)

- Calories: 70
- Fat: 5g
- Carbs: 8g

- Fiber: 4g
- Sugar: 3g
- Protein: 2g

78. ZUCCHINI CHIPS (OVEN-BAKED)

Prep Time: 10 Mins

Cook Time: 20-25 Mins

Total Time: 30-35 Mins

Servings: 4

Ingredients

- 2 medium zucchinis, thinly Sliced
- 1 tbsp olive oil
- 1 tsp garlic powder
- 1 tsp dried oregano
- ½tsp sea salt
- ¼ tsp black pepper

Instructions

1. Put parchment paper on a baking pan and preheat the oven to 400°F (200°C).
2. Using a sharp knife or mandoline slicer, cut the zucchini into thin rounds approximately ⅛ inches thick.
3. Toss the zucchini slices in a large bowl with salt, pepper, oregano, olive oil, and garlic powder until they are uniformly coated.
4. Arrange the zucchini slices in a single layer on the prepared baking sheet, being careful not to overlap.
5. Bake the zucchini chips for 20 to 25 minutes, turning them over halfway through, or until they are crispy and golden.
6. Before serving, let them cool for a few minutes.

Notes

- ✓ Be sure to slice the zucchini evenly to ensure consistent cooking.
- ✓ If you want extra crispiness, leave the chips in the oven for a few more minutes, but watch them closely to prevent burning.

Nutrition Info (Per Serving)

- Calories: 60
- Fat: 4g

- Carbs: 7g
- Fiber: 2g
- Sugar: 4g
- Protein: 2g

79 CABBAGE STEAKS WITH GARLIC

Prep Time: 10 Mins

Cook Time: 25 Mins

Total Time: 35 Mins

Servings: 4

Ingredients

- 1 medium head of cabbage
- 2 tbsp olive oil
- 4 cloves garlic, chop-up
- ½tsp sea salt
- ¼ tsp black pepper
- 1 tbsp lemon juice (non-compulsory)

Instructions

1. Put parchment paper on a baking pan and preheat the oven to 400°F (200°C).
2. Cut the cabbage into steaks that are 1 inch thick after removing the outer leaves.
3. Place the cabbage steaks on the baking sheet.
4. Sprinkle the cabbage with salt and pepper, and chop up garlic after drizzling it with olive oil.
5. Bake the cabbage for 20 to 25 minutes, turning it halfway through, or until it is soft and has a faint browning around the edges.
6. Before serving, drizzle with fresh lemon juice, if desired.

Notes

- ✓ For extra flavor, you can top the cabbage steaks with fresh herbs such as thyme or rosemary.
- ✓ These make a great side dish for any main course.

Nutrition Info (Per Serving)

- Calories: 100
- Fat: 7g
- Carbs: 11g

- Fiber: 5g
- Sugar: 5g
- Protein: 3g

80. ROASTED ARTICHOKE HEARTS

Prep Time: 5 Mins

Cook Time: 25-30 Mins

Total Time: 30-35 Mins

Servings: 4

Ingredients

- 4 artichoke hearts (fresh or jarred in water, drained)
- 2 tbsp olive oil
- 1 tsp dried thyme
- ½tsp sea salt
- ¼ tsp black pepper
- 1 tbsp lemon juice (non-compulsory)

Instructions

1. Preheat the oven to 400°F (200°C) and line a baking sheet with parchment paper.
2. Cut the artichoke hearts in half (if using whole) and place them on the baking sheet.
3. Drizzle with olive oil and sprinkle with thyme, salt, and pepper.
4. Roast in the oven for 25-30 min, flipping halfway through, until the artichokes are golden and crispy on the edges.
5. Non-compulsory: Drizzle with fresh lemon juice before serving.

Notes

- ✓ These roasted artichokes can be served as a snack or side dish. They're also great with a dipping sauce like tahini or a lemon garlic sauce.
- ✓ If using jarred artichokes, make sure they're well-drained before roasting.

Nutrition Info (Per Serving)

- Calories: 120
- Fat: 10g
- Carbs: 10g
- Fiber: 6g

- Sugar: 2g
- Protein: 3g

81. COCONUT MILK PANNA COTTA

Prep Time: 10 Mins

Cook Time: 5 Mins

Total Time: 4 Hrs (Including Chilling)

Servings: 4

Ingredients

- 1 can (13.5 oz) full-fat coconut milk
- 2 tbsp water
- 1½tsp grass-fed gelatin powder
- 1 ½tbsp stevia (or adjust+)
- 1 tsp vanilla extract
- Pinch of sea salt

Instructions

1. Sprinkle the gelatin over the water in a small bowl and leave it for five min to bloom.
2. Heat the coconut milk in a saucepan over medium heat until it begins to steam, but do not bring it to a boil.
3. Add stevia, vanilla, and a dash of salt to the coconut milk. Mix to blend.
4. Please remove the heat and whisk the bloomed gelatin until it dissolves completely.
5. Transfer the blend into little glasses or ramekins.
6. Set in the refrigerator for at least 4 hrs.
7. Serve cold. Non-compulsory garnishes include unsweetened shredded coconut or a few fresh berries if tolerated.

Notes

- ✓ For a softer panna cotta, use slightly less gelatin.
- ✓ For a firmer texture, add an extra ½tsp gelatin.
- ✓ Make sure the coconut milk is full-fat for best results.

Nutrition Info (Per Serving)

- Calories: 180

- Fat: 18g
- Carbs: 3g
- Sugar: 1g
- Protein: 3g

82. CINNAMON ALMOND BUTTER BALLS

Total Time: 10 Mins

Servings: 12

Ingredients

- 1 cup of almond butter (smooth)
- ¼ cup of unsweetened shredded coconut
- 1 tsp cinnamon
- 2 tbsp coconut flour
- 1 tbsp chia seeds (non-compulsory)
- 1-2 tbsp stevia or monk fruit sweetener (as needed)

Instructions

1. Almond butter, shredded coconut, cinnamon, coconut flour, chia seeds, and sweetener should all be mixed in a large bowl.
2. Mix everything until it takes on the consistency of thick dough.
3. Make 12 balls of the same size by rolling the dough.
4. Arrange the balls on a parchment paper-lined plate or baking sheet.
5. Before serving, let it firm up in the refrigerator for at least half an hr.

Notes

- ✓ If the dough is too sticky to form balls, add more coconut flour, 1 tsp, until the desired consistency is revealed.
- ✓ You can also roll these balls in extra shredded coconut or ground cinnamon for added texture.

Nutrition Info (Per Serving)

- Calories: 150
- Fat: 12g
- Carbs: 6g
- Fiber: 3g
- Sugar: 1g
- protein: 5g

83. COCONUT FLOUR BROWNIES (NO SUGAR)

Prep Time: 10 Mins

Cook Time: 20-25 Mins

Total Time: 30-35 Mins

Servings: 9

Ingredients

- ½cup of coconut flour
- ¼ cup of unsweetened cocoa powder
- ¼ cup of coconut oil, melted
- 4 large eggs
- ½cup of stevia or monk fruit sweetener
- 1 tsp vanilla extract
- ¼ tsp sea salt
- ½tsp baking powder

Instructions

1. Put parchment paper into a 9 × 9-inch baking pan and preheat the oven to 350°F (175°C).
2. Mix the baking powder, sea salt, cocoa powder, and coconut flour in a medium-sized bowl.
3. Beat the eggs, sweetener, vanilla extract, and melted coconut oil in a separate dish until creamy.
4. Stir the dry and wet components together until they are thoroughly blended.
5. Evenly distribute the brownie mixture after pouring it into the prepared pan.
6. A toothpick inserted in the center should come out clean after 20 to 25 min of baking.
7. Before dividing the brownies into nine squares and serving, let them cool.

Notes

✓ These brownies are rich and dense. For a lighter texture, you can add ¼ cups of unsweetened almond milk.
✓ Non-compulsory: Add chop-up dark chocolate or walnuts for extra flavor.

Nutrition Info (Per Serving)

- Calories: 180
- Fat: 15g

- Carbs: 6g
- Fiber: 4g
- Protein: 6g

84. AVOCADO CHOCOLATE MOUSSE (WITH STEVIA)

Total Time: 5 Mins

Servings: 4

Ingredients

- 2 ripe avocados, peeled and pitted
- ¼ cup of unsweetened cocoa powder
- ¼ cup of almond milk (or any unsweetened milk)
- 1 tsp vanilla extract
- 2 tbsp stevia or monk fruit sweetener (adjust+)
- Pinch of sea salt

Instructions

1. Put the avocados, stevia, almond milk, chocolate powder, vanilla extract, and salt in a blender or food processor.
2. Blend till creamy and smooth.
3. If necessary, add additional stevia or your preferred sweetener after tasting.
4. Before serving, spoon the mousse into serving dishes and let it sit in the refrigerator for at least an hr.
5. Garnish with a dollop of whipped coconut cream or fresh berries for added richness.

Notes

- ✓ This mousse can be made of time and stored in the fridge for up to 2 days.
- ✓ Add a pinch of cinnamon or a few drops of peppermint extract for a flavor twist.

Nutrition Info (Per Serving)

- Calories: 160
- Fat: 14g
- Carbs: 10g
- Fiber: 7g
- Sugar: 1g
- Protein: 2g

85. LEMON COCONUT BARS

Prep Time: 10 Mins

Cook Time: 20 Mins

Total Time: 30 Mins

Servings: 8

Ingredients

- 1 cup of unsweetened shredded coconut
- ½cup of coconut flour
- ¼ cup of coconut oil, melted
- ¼ cup of fresh lemon juice
- 1 tbsp lemon zest
- 2 large eggs
- 1 tbsp stevia or monk fruit sweetener
- ½tsp vanilla extract
- Pinch of sea salt

Instructions

1. Put parchment paper into an 8 × 8-inch baking pan and preheat the oven to 350°F (175°C).
2. Add the salt, coconut flour, and shredded coconut to a large mixing basin.
3. Whisk together the eggs, sweetener, vanilla extract, lemon juice, lemon zest, and melted coconut oil in a separate dish.
4. Stir the dry ingredients with the liquid components until they are well blended.
5. Evenly distribute the batter after pouring it into the baking pan.
6. Bake the bars for 18 to 20 min or until they are firm and golden brown.
7. Before cutting the bars into eight squares and serving, let them cool fully.

Notes

- ✓ These bars can be stored in an airtight container in the refrigerator for up to 5 days.
- ✓ You can add a little extra lemon zest for an extra citrus kick.

Nutrition Info (Per Serving)

- Calories: 200
- Fat: 18g
- Carbs: 6g

- Fiber: 3g
- Sugar: 2g
- Protein: 4g

86. PALEO PUMPKIN PIE (NO SWEETENER)

Prep Time: 10 Mins

Cook Time: 40 Mins

Total Time: 50 Mins

Servings: 8

Ingredients

- 1½cup of pumpkin puree (preferably homemade or organic)
- 3 large eggs
- ½cup of full-fat coconut milk
- 1 tsp ground cinnamon
- ½tsp ground ginger
- ¼ tsp ground nutmeg
- ¼ tsp ground cloves
- ¼ tsp sea salt
- 1 tsp vanilla extract
- ½cup of almond flour (for crust)

Instructions

1. Set the oven's temperature to 175°C (350°F).
2. Mix the pumpkin puree, eggs, coconut milk, cloves, nutmeg, ginger, cinnamon, and sea salt in a medium bowl and whisk until smooth and thoroughly blended.
3. On a pie plate, pour the pumpkin mixture.
4. Mix the almond flour and vanilla essence in a separate dish to make a crumbly dough. Press the mixture into the bottom of the pie plate to form a crust.
5. A toothpick placed into the center of the pie should come out clean after 35 to 40 min of baking, which is when the filling is set.
6. Before serving, allow the pie to cool thoroughly.

Notes

- ✓ This pie can be made over time and stored in the fridge for up to 4 days.
- ✓ Top the pie with a dollop of whipped coconut cream before serving for extra texture.

Nutrition Info (Per Serving)

- Calories: 170
- Fat: 14g
- Carbs: 10g
- Fiber: 3g
- Sugar: 4g
- Protein: 4g

87. CHIA COCONUT FAT BOMBS

Total Time: 5 Mins

Servings: 10

Ingredients

- ½cup of coconut oil, melted
- ¼ cup of unsweetened shredded coconut
- ¼ cup of chia seeds
- 1 tbsp coconut flour
- ½tsp vanilla extract
- Stevia or monk fruit sweetener (as needed)

Instructions

1. Melted coconut oil, shredded coconut, chia seeds, coconut flour, and vanilla essence should all be mixed in a small bowl.
2. Stir thoroughly until the chia seeds absorb the coconut oil and everything is mixed.
3. Spoon the mixture into tiny muffin pans or silicone molds.
4. Freeze until solid, at least 1 hr.
5. Remove the fat bombs from the molds and place them in an airtight container in the freezer.

Notes

- ✓ These fat bombs are rich in healthy fats and are perfect for a quick energy boost.
- ✓ You can adjust the sweetness by adding more or less stevia or monk fruit sweetener.

Nutrition Info (Per Serving)

- Calories: 120
- Fat: 12g

- Carbs: 3g
- Fiber: 3g
- Sugar: 1g
- Protein: 2g

88. CINNAMON VANILLA CHIA PUDDING

Prep Time: 5 Mins

Total Time: 4 Hrs

Servings: 4

Ingredients

- 1 cup of unsweetened almond milk (or any preferred milk)
- ½cup of chia seeds
- 1 tsp cinnamon
- 1 tsp vanilla extract
- 1-2 tbsp stevia or monk fruit sweetener (as needed)

Instructions

1. Combine the almond milk, chia seeds, cinnamon, vanilla extract, and sweetener in a medium-sized bowl and whisk to combine.
2. Please ensure the chia seeds are thoroughly mixed with the liquid by
3. stirring in the bowl and refrigerating for at least four hours or overnight. This will enable the chia seeds to absorb the liquid and develop a pudding-like consistency.
4. Serve cold. Non-compulsory: Before serving, garnish with cinnamon or fresh berries.

Notes

- ✓ If you prefer a smoother consistency, blend the chia pudding in a blender after it has been set for a few minutes.
- ✓ The pudding can be stored in the refrigerator for up to 4 days.

Nutrition Info (Per Serving)

- Calories: 100
- Fat: 7g
- Carbs: 8g
- Fiber: 7g
- Sugar: 1g
- Protein: 3g

89. BAKED CINNAMON APPLES (SMALL AMOUNTS IF TOLERATED)

Prep Time: 10 Mins

Cook Time: 25-30 Mins

Total Time: 35-40 Mins

Servings: 4

Ingredients

- 4 medium apples (such as Granny Smith)
- 1 tsp ground cinnamon
- 1 tbsp coconut oil, melted
- 1 tbsp stevia or monk fruit sweetener (non-compulsory)
- ¼ cup of unsweetened apple cider (or water)

Instructions

1. Preheat the oven to 350°F (175°C) and grease a baking dish with coconut oil.

2. Create a well in the middle of the apples for the filling by cooking them.
3. Mix the cinnamon, melted coconut oil, and sweetener (if using) in a small bowl.
4. Fill the middle of the baking dish with the cinnamon mixture after placing the apples inside.
5. Cover the apples in the dish with apple cider (or water).
6. Bake for 25 to 30 min, or until the apples are soft, covered with aluminum foil.
7. Warm up and serve. Add a dollop of coconut cream or a sprinkling of cinnamon for added taste.

Notes

- ✓ If the apples are too tart, you can adjust the sweetness+ with the stevia or monk fruit sweetener.
- ✓ Use apples lower in sugar, such as Granny Smith, for a more tart flavor.

Nutrition Info (Per Serving)

- Calories: 100
- Fat: 5g
- Carbs: 19g
- Fiber: 4g
- Sugar: 12g

90. TURMERIC COCONUT ICE CREAM (STEVIA-SWEETENED)

Total Time: 10 Mins

Servings: 6

Ingredients

- 1 can (14 oz) full-fat coconut milk
- ½cup of coconut cream (for extra richness)
- 1 tsp ground turmeric
- 1 tsp vanilla extract
- 1 tbsp stevia or monk fruit sweetener (adjust+)
- Pinch of black pepper (non-compulsory to enhance turmeric absorption)

Instructions

1. Mix the coconut milk, coconut cream, stevia, turmeric, vanilla extract, and black pepper (if using) in a mixing bowl and whisk until smooth and thoroughly blended.
2. Fill an ice cream machine with the ingredients and churn for 20 to 25 min, as the manufacturer directs.
3. Transfer the churned ice cream to a container and freeze it for at least two hrs or until it solidifies.
4. Serve right away for a soft-serve consistency; for a harder texture, freeze for a longer period of time.

Notes

- ✓ If you don't have an ice cream maker, you can pour the mixture into a shallow dish and freeze, stirring every 30 minutes for 2-3 hours to break up ice crystals.
- ✓ Turmeric has a naturally strong flavor, so adjust the amount to your taste preferences.

Nutrition Info (Per Serving)

- Calories: 180
- Fat: 18g
- Carbs: 6g
- Fiber: 3g
- Sugar: 1g
- Protein: 1g

91. GINGEKR LEMON HERBAL TEA

Prep Time: 5 Mins

Cook Time: 5 Mins

Total Time: 10 Mins

Servings: 1

Ingredients

- 1-inch piece of fresh ginger root, peeled and Sliced thin
- 1 tbsp fresh lemon juice
- 1 tsp stevia or monk fruit sweetener (non-compulsory)
- 2 cups of hot water
- 1-2 lemon slices (non-compulsory for garnish)

Instructions

1. In a small saucepan, bring 2 cups of water to a boil.
2. After adding the Sliced ginger to the boiling water, reduce the heat to a simmer.
3. After letting the ginger simmer for around five min, turn off the heat.
4. Pour the tea through a strainer into a cup and mix with the sugar (if using) and fresh lemon juice.
5. If preferred, garnish with slices of lemon and serve hot.

Notes

- ✓ Ginger is known for its digestive benefits and is often used in candida diets for its anti-inflammatory properties.
- ✓ You can add more ginger or let it steep for a longer time for a stronger ginger flavor.

Nutrition Info (Per Serving)

- Calories: 5
- Fat: 0g
- Carbs: 1g
- Fiber: 0g
- Sugar: 1g
- Protein: 0g

92. CINNAMON COCONUT MILK LATTE

Prep Time: 5 Mins

Cook Time: 5 Mins

Total Time: 10 Mins

Servings: 1

Ingredients

- 1 cup of full-fat coconut milk (or your preferred milk)
- ½tsp ground cinnamon
- 1 tsp vanilla extract
- 1 tsp stevia or monk fruit sweetener (non-compulsory)
- ½cup of brewed coffee or espresso (non-compulsory for a caffeine boost)

Instructions

1. Heat the coconut milk in a small saucepan over medium heat until it's warm (but not boiling).
2. Add the cinnamon, vanilla extract, and sweetener (if using) to the milk and whisk until fully incorporated.
3. If using coffee or espresso, pour it into your mug.
4. Pour the cinnamon-coconut milk mixture into the mug with the coffee (or just the coconut milk if you're not using coffee).
5. Stir and serve hot. Non-compulsoryly, sprinkle a little extra cinnamon on top.

Notes

- ✓ For a frothy texture, use a milk frother or whisk the milk vigorously before serving.
- ✓ This drink can be made with any plant-based milk, but coconut milk provides a rich, creamy texture that complements the cinnamon flavor.

Nutrition Info (Per Serving)

- Calories: 120
- Fat: 11g
- Carbs: 3g
- Fiber: 2g
- Sugar: 1g
- Protein: 1g

93. CUCUMBER MINT DETOX WATER

Total Time: 5 Mins

Servings: 4

Ingredients

- ½cucumber, Thinly Sliced
- ¼ cup of fresh mint leaves
- 1 lemon, thinly Sliced
- 4 cups of filtered water
- Ice cubes (non-compulsory)

Instructions

1. Mix the cucumber slices, fresh mint leaves, and lemon slices in a large pitcher.
2. Add the filtered water and stir to mix.
3. Let the water infuse in the refrigerator for at least 1-2 hrs (or overnight for a stronger flavor).
4. Serve chilled, with ice cubes if desired.

Notes

- ✓ This refreshing drink is perfect for detoxifying and hydrating your body.
- ✓ You can reuse the cucumber, lemon, and mint slices for another batch of water.

Nutrition Info (Per Serving)

- Calories: 5
- Carbs: 1g
- Sugar: 1g

94. ALOE VERA GUT HEALING DRINK

Total Time: 5 Mins

Servings: 1

Ingredients

- ¼ cup of fresh aloe vera gel (or 100% pure aloe vera juice)
- 1 cup of filtered water
- 1 tsp lemon juice
- 1 tsp stevia or monk fruit sweetener (non-compulsory)
- Pinch of sea salt (non-compulsory)

Instructions

1. If using fresh aloe vera gel, carefully extract it from the aloe leaf by cutting off the outer skin and scraping it with a spoon.
2. In a blender, mix the aloe vera gel (or aloe juice), water, lemon juice, sweetener (if using), and a pinch of sea salt (if desired).
3. Blend until smooth and healthy mixed.
4. Serve immediately or store in the refrigerator for up to 24 hrs.

Notes

✓ Aloe vera is known for its soothing properties, which can help support digestion and gut health.
✓ Fresh aloe vera gel can be difficult to find, so substitute it with high-quality aloe vera juice.

Nutrition Info (Per Serving)

- Calories: 15
- Carbs: 4
- Fiber: 1g
- Sugar: 2g

95. APPLE CIDER VINEGAR TONIC

Total Time: 5 Minsk

Servings: 1

Ingredients

- 1 tbsp organic apple cider vinegar (with the "mother")
- 1 cup of warm filtered water
- ½tsp cinnamon (non-compulsory)
- 1 tsp stevia or monk fruit sweetener (non-compulsory)
- 1 tsp fresh lemon juice (non-compulsory)

Instructions

1. In a cup, mix the warm water and apple cider vinegar.
2. Stir in the cinnamon, sweetener, and lemon juice (if using).
3. Mix well until everything is dissolved.
4. Drink immediately while warm, or chill it for a cold tonic.

Notes

✓ Apple cider vinegar has several health benefits, including promoting digestion and supporting blood sugar balance.
✓ You can adjust the apple cider vinegar and sweetener amount based on your preferences.

Nutrition Info (Per Serving)

- Calories: 5
- Carbs: 1g
- Sugar: 1g

96. TURMERIC GOLDEN MILK (UNSWEETENED)

Prep Time: 5 Mins

Cook Time: 5 Mins

Total Time: 10 Mins

Servings: 1

Ingredients

- 1 cup of unsweetened almond milk (or other dairy-free milk)
- ½tsp ground turmeric
- ¼ tsp ground cinnamon
- ¼ tsp ground ginger
- Pinch of black pepper (to enhance turmeric absorption)
- 1 tsp coconut oil (non-compulsory for creaminess)
- ¼ tsp vanilla extract (non-compulsory)

Instructions

1. Warm (but not boiling) the almond milk in a small saucepan over medium heat.
2. Add the black pepper, ginger, cinnamon, turmeric, and coconut oil (if using).
3. Stir until the coconut oil has melted and all the spices have been well mixed.
4. For added taste, pour the mixture into a cup and, if using, add vanilla essence.
5. Mix and savor warm.

Notes

✓ Turmeric contains curcumin, which is known for its anti-inflammatory properties.
✓ You can adjust the sweetness with stevia or monk fruit sweetener if desired.

Nutrition Info (Per Serving)

- Calories: 50
- Fat: 4g
- Carbs: 2g
- Fiber: 1g
- Protein: 1g

97. FENNEL AND GINGER TEA

Prep Time: 5 Mins

Cook Time: 5 Mins

Total Time: 10 Mins

Servings: 1

Ingredients

- 1 tsp fennel seeds
- 1-inch piece of fresh ginger, Sliced
- 1 cup of filtered water
- 1 tsp lemon juice (non-compulsory)
- 1 tsp stevia or monk fruit sweetener (non-compulsory)

Instructions

1. Put the water, fresh ginger slices, and fennel seeds in a small saucepan.
2. After bringing it to a boil, lower the heat to a simmer and steep for five
3. minutes.
4. Add lemon juice and sweetener after straining the tea into a cup if desired.
5. Mix and savor warm.

Notes

✓ Fennel and ginger are both great for digestion and can help reduce bloating.
✓ You can store the fennel seeds in an airtight container for future use.

Nutrition Info (Per Serving)

- Calories: 5
- Carbs: 1g
- Fiber: 1g

98. PEPPERMINT TEA

Prep Time: 2 Mins

Cook Time: 5 Mins

Total Time: 7 Mins

Servings: 1

Ingredients

- 1-2 tsp dried peppermint leaves (or one peppermint tea bag)
- 1 cup of boiling water
- 1 tsp stevia or monk fruit sweetener (non-compulsory)

Instructions

1. Put the tea bag or dried peppermint leaves in a cup.
2. Cover the peppermint with the boiling water.
3. After around five minutes of steeping, strain the leaves or remove the tea bag.
4. If preferred, stir in sugar and serve hot. Put the tea bag or dried peppermint leaves in a cup.
5. Cover the peppermint with the boiling water.
6. After around five minutes of steeping, strain the leaves or remove the tea bag.
7. If preferred, stir in sugar and serve hot.

Notes

- ✓ Peppermint tea is naturally soothing and can help digestion, especially after meals.
- ✓ If available, you can make this tea with fresh peppermint leaves, using about 2-3 sprigs.

Nutrition Info (Per Serving)

- ↓ Calories: 2
- ↓ Carbs: 1g

99. GREEN TEA WITH LEMON

Prep Time: 2 Mins

Cook Time: 3 Mins

Total Time: 5 Mins

Ingredients

- 1 green tea bag (or 1 tsp loose-leaf green tea)
- 1 cup of boiling water
- 1 tbsp fresh lemon juice
- 1 tsp stevia or monk fruit sweetener (non-compulsory)

Instructions

1. Place the green tea bag or loose-leaf tea in a cup.
2. Pour the boiling water over the tea and let it steep for 2-3 min.
3. Remove the tea bag or strain the loose leaves.
4. Stir in fresh lemon juice and sweetener (if using).
5. Serve warm and enjoy.

Notes

- ✓ Green tea is known for its antioxidant properties and is a great metabolism booster.
- ✓ Depending on your preference, you can adjust the steeping time for a lighter or stronger flavor.

Nutrition Info (Per Serving)

- Calories: 5
- Carbs: 1g

100. BONE BROTH SMOOTHIE (SAVORY)

Total Time: 5 Mins

Servings: 1

Ingredients

- 1 cup of high-quality bone broth (chilled or slightly warm, but not hot)
- ½ small avocado
- ½ cup of baby spinach
- 1 tbsp fresh lemon juice
- 1 tbsp collagen peptides (non-compulsory for extra protein)
- 1 tbsp olive oil or MCT oil
- ½ tsp sea salt
- ¼ tsp black pepper

- Non-compulsory: pinch of turmeric or ginger powder for extra anti-inflammatory benefits

Instructions
1. Put everything in a blender.
2. Blend until smooth and creamy.
3. If necessary, taste and adjust the seasoning.
4. Pour into a glass and start drinking right away!

Notes
- ✓ If you prefer a thinner texture, add a few tbsp of extra bone broth or a splash of water.
- ✓ Use chilled bone broth if you like cold or lightly warmed broth if you prefer a cozy drink.
- ✓ Great as a healing, nutrient-dense breakfast or snack.

Nutrition Info (Per Serving)

- Calories: 250
- Fat: 22g
- Carbs: 5g
- Fiber: 3g
- Sugar: 1g
- Protein: 10g

THE END

Printed in Dunstable, United Kingdom

67049696R00060